Skills in Neighbourhood Work

Skills in Neighbourhood Work is a practice textbook. It explains the skills, knowledge and techniques needed by community workers and other practitioners to work effectively in and with communities.

While the principles and methods it describes have stood the test of time, the political, economic and social changes which have taken place since the book was first published have made new editions essential. Rewritten and updated to include new practice examples, this fifth edition retains all the practical information needed by the student or practitioner but sets it in the contemporary context. Including a European perspective and views from North America and Australia, it covers:

Starting, supporting and ending work with community groups
Evaluation
Data collection
Goals and priorities
Making contacts
Group work
Helping groups work with other organisations

This invaluable textbook is essential reading for students and practitioners of community work.

Paul Henderson and **David N. Thomas** have worked in community development since the early 1970s. Their experience includes neighbourhood work, training, consultancy and research. Most recently, they worked together as directors at the Community Development Foundation. They have also published extensively, in both the United Kingdom and mainland Europe.

Skills in Neighbourhood Work

5th Edition

Paul Henderson and David N. Thomas

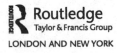
Routledge
Taylor & Francis Group

LONDON AND NEW YORK

Cover image: Peaceful protest in downtown Kansas City © Getty Images

Fifth edition published 2023
by Routledge
4 Park Square, Milton Park, Abingdon, Oxon, OX14 4RN

and by Routledge
605 Third Avenue, New York, NY 10158

Routledge is an imprint of the Taylor & Francis Group, an informa business

© 2023 **Paul Henderson and David N. Thomas**

First edition published by Unwin Hyman Ltd 1980

Fourth edition published by Routledge 2013

British Library Cataloguing-in-Publication Data
A catalogue record for this book is available from the British Library

Library of Congress Cataloging-in-Publication Data
Names: Henderson, Paul, author. | Thomas, David N., 1945– author.
Title: Skills in neighbourhood work / Paul Henderson and David N. Thomas.
Description: 5th Edition. | New York, NY : Routledge, 2023. | Revised edition
  of the authors' Skills in neighbourhood work, 2013. | Includes bibliographical
  references and index.
Identifiers: LCCN 2022036580 (print) | LCCN 2022036581 (ebook) | ISBN
  9781032314921 (hardback) | ISBN 9781032314600 (paperback) | ISBN
  9781003310006 (ebook)
Subjects: LCSH: Social group work—Great Britain. | Community organization—
  Great Britain.
Classification: LCC HV245 .H396 2023 (print) | LCC HV245 (ebook) |
  DDC 361.40941—dc23/eng/20220818
LC record available at https://lccn.loc.gov/2022036580
LC ebook record available at https://lccn.loc.gov/2022036581

ISBN: 978-1-032-31492-1 (hbk)
ISBN: 978-1-032-31460-0 (pbk)
ISBN: 978-1-003-31000-6 (ebk)

DOI: 10.4324/9781003310006

Typeset in Sabon
by Apex CoVantage, LLC

To community development friends in Europe

Contents

Figures

Tables

Acknowledgements

The writing of this book over 40 years ago was achieved through collaboration with many people in the United Kingdom and the rest of Europe.

We owe a considerable debt to those practitioners to whom we were consultants and to those who participated in a series of workshops on neighbourhood work skills. The workshops ran for half a day a week over five weeks. The participants were community workers from London and the south. We encouraged participants not only to describe their practice but also to role-play particular experiences – a memorable example was a community worker in south London entering a betting shop in order to make contact with local people.

We developed the contents of each chapter in these workshops and in seminars at the National Institute for Social work (NISW), London, during the 1970s. NISW specialised in post-professional education and training. We were community work lecturers, having previously been practitioners. We could not have produced the book without the help of Jacki Reason at NISW. She was a continuing source of patience, support and hard work on this and other projects. We also acknowledge the help and encouragement of visiting American colleagues, including Harry Specht, Ralph Kramer, Jack Rothman and Charlie Grosser.

There have been five translations of the book. Our thanks to Ad Raspe, then of the Netherlands Institute for Community Development, whose hard work led to the Dutch translation of the book, and to Maryse Pegourie and Hugo Swinnen who organised the French translation. We are grateful to Anneke Touwen in the Netherlands for initiating translations of the third edition into Slovakian and Croatian. A translation into Polish was agreed in 2012.

The second edition (1987) was made possible by grants from the Wates and Barings foundations, and we are grateful for their support. Again, we were helped in preparing this edition by a number of practitioners and trainers, this time from several countries, who responded to our request for help in revising the book.

The third edition (2002) involved a more major revision of the text. It was made possible by grants from the Joseph Rowntree Charitable Trust and Lloyds TSB Foundation for England and Wales and the support of the Community Development Foundation (CDF). We also involved practitioners and trainers in providing new material. In particular, we wish to thank Marjorie Mayo (Goldsmiths College, University of London), Tor Justad (consultant) and Yvette Smalle (Leeds Beckett University) who gave advice and suggestions on, respectively, the issues of women and community development, community economic development and race in the context of neighbourhood work; Ruth Stewart (Rural Community Network, Northern Ireland), Fiona Ballantyne (Inverclyde Council), Yvette Smalle and Gerard Hautekeur (Flemish national community development organisation) who all sent us practice examples; and Ad Raspe (Verwey-Jonker Institute), Alan Barr (Scottish Community Development Centre), Alison Gilchrist, Gabriel Chanan, Kevin Harris (all of CDF) and Marjorie Mayo for commenting on the introductory chapter. Ilona Vercseg (Hungarian Association for Community Development) and Hans Andersson and Viveca Urwitz in Sweden provided encouragement and support throughout.

The updating of the book for a fourth edition (2013) was prompted by our awareness of the economic, political and social changes, which had taken place over the previous ten years – with their inevitable impact on community development and neighbourhood work. Our publisher and colleagues encouraged us to bring the book up to date and their enthusiasm was invaluable. So too was that of our families: Stevie, Danny and Sian; and Barbara, Juliet, Jamie and Barney.

During the time that we prepared the fourth edition, we owed a special debt of gratitude to Alison Gilchrist and Stuart Hashagen. As community development consultants and trainers, they were able to make valuable suggestions for updating our material. Alison advised us on how to strengthen equalities issues in the book, and Stuart provided a Scottish perspective and drafted the new chapter on evaluation and the appendix. Responsibility, however, rests with us alone.

Continuing interest in the book led us and our publisher to proceed with this edition. It has involved a major revision of Chapter 1 and the insertion of new examples and some updating in the other chapters. These were sent to us by longstanding friends and former colleagues, and our gratitude to them is immense. We hope the end result will be of help to those people who are directly involved, in one capacity or another, in neighbourhood work.

We are grateful to Routledge for having suggested this edition and to Claire Jarvis and Sully Evans for managing it.

1 Key ideas about neighbourhood work

We have written this book to help those working in neighbourhoods. It is intended for people who, in one form or another, practise community-level work as a paid job. It is also for those who use its principles and methods as part of another profession, such as economic development or health. We also hope that it will help local people tackle needs and issues that affect their livelihoods, quality of life and the neighbourhood. The potential readers can be specified as follows:

- community development workers, especially those working in neighbourhoods;
- students on training courses (qualifying and post-qualifying) that include input on neighbourhood work, for example, youth and community work courses, applied social studies, and planning and economic development courses;
- regeneration officers, planners and staff involved in cross-sectoral partnerships on economic, social and environmental programmes;
- other practitioners who make use of neighbourhood work skills and methods as a significant part of their jobs, for example, youth workers, housing officers, public health workers, rural development staff and community arts workers;
- managers, especially those with responsibility for community-based regeneration and community planning programmes;
- community leaders who are key members of community groups and networks;
- 'unpaid' community workers: local people experienced in community action who take on the role of the community worker.

This chapter will place neighbourhood work in the wider context of community development, and we will relate *Skills in Neighbourhood Work* to the community development literature. We will then put forward key changes which mean that the idea of neighbourhood needs to be updated. The changes are examined in three ways:

- Changes in people's experiences of neighbourhood
- The extent to which neighbourhoods have changed
- The impact of the COVID-19 pandemic, Black Lives Matter, climate change and Brexit on neighbourhood work

We suggest why strengthening communities at neighbourhood level remains of central importance for society. The chapter ends with an explanation of how we conceive of neighbourhood work as a process or series of stages.

DOI: 10.4324/9781003310006-1

The identification of themes, issues and concepts has been carried out, for the most part, with a United Kingdom (UK) focus although we shall see that many of the themes are echoed in other countries and cultures. Within the United Kingdom, there are significant differences of governance in both the formulation and application of policies. Equally, there are important differences in England, Scotland, Wales and Northern Ireland in the practice of working with communities. We have sought to reflect these differences in the examples we have selected. Our approach to the updating has been to seek recent and current examples of practice that illustrate particular skills and roles and to delete references to publications known to be out of print or difficult to access. Page number references are included for publications which are easily available but not for the older, less accessible material.

The language surrounding the methods, purposes and values of working with communities has changed significantly over the years – and no doubt will continue to change. This presents a challenge. There are no quick and easy answers to the question 'what is neighbourhood work?' and 'what is community development?' Similarly there are inherent difficulties with the concept of community, an idea with which sociologists and others have wrestled for many years and which, in day-to-day life, is used with many different meanings.

We use 'neighbourhood work' to refer to direct face-to-face work with local people who form groups, organisations and networks to tackle a need or problem they have identified, to give support to each other and/or provide services to local people in the area. While the term is not as widely used as it was in the past, we have chosen to retain it to describe close, supportive work with people committed to their community. We do not wish to give neighbourhood work a wholly geographical definition. Just because workers are engaged primarily at neighbourhood level, it does not mean that they cannot or should not be actively involved with wider concerns, whether these be city-wide, national or international. The overriding focus for interventions by neighbourhood practitioners entails working closely with neighbourhood-based groups. Supporting groups that share a common interest or identity across a wider area occupies less of a worker's time.

The terms neighbourhood work and community work both refer to how a practitioner works with local people. They are terms which are about skills, methods and values and about engaging with communities. Community work is a more generic concept than neighbourhood work (and is used in a variety of contexts). Community development is used to refer to the processes of change and learning that take place in communities. Most people also refer to the community development profession. The term neighbourhood work suggests to us a job for which a range of explicit, hard skills are required in order to work effectively and sensitively with local people. Local people want the service and support of skilled professional practitioners, just as they want, for example, skilled midwives, skilled caretakers and skilled plumbers. It is important to convey the tangible, practical content of working with local people. 'Neighbourhood work' does this. Essentially, the description of neighbourhood work skills as set out in this volume seeks to answer the question *'how to do it?'* The book does not take forward a discussion *about* neighbourhood work or community development or about 'community'. We are concerned with the laying out of 'know-how' propositions. Implicit in this approach is a requirement to specify the series of tasks that are involved.

Community development literature

When the first edition of this book was published, it was one of only a few texts available to help practitioners and students to be more effective neighbourhood workers. This is no longer the case. There have been a number of further contributions to the practice theory of neighbourhood work: Twelvetrees (2008), Smith (1994), Barr (1996), Wilson and Wilde (2001), Richardson (2008), Pitchford (2008), and Gilchrist (2019) and – a new development in the 1990s – books on rural community work by Francis and Henderson (1992) and Derounian (1998). The amount of material suggesting ways of finding out about a neighbourhood has grown, for example Hawtin and Percy-Smith (2007), as have guides on participation methods and community engagement (New Economics Foundation, 1998).

One reason for the expansion of the skills literature was the stimulus provided by the regeneration programmes of the 1997–2010 Labour government. Its national strategy for neighbourhood renewal in England sought to put residents at the heart of regeneration. It also aimed to broaden and strengthen neighbourhood renewal skills amongst a variety of professionals and practitioners (Department for Communities and Local Government (DCLG), 2002). The latter publication was followed by the *Egan Review* (Egan, 2004), which examined the skills and knowledge needed for sustainable communities work. There were no equivalent publications during the subsequent Conservative administration, not surprisingly given the austerity policy and cuts to national community development organisations (Community Development Exchange closed in 2012, the Community Development Foundation in 2016 and the Federation of Community Development Learning in 2017). David Cameron's 'Big Society' initiative in 2010 promised community involvement but very little happened on the ground and certainly nothing was added to the skills literature. The prime minister had asked Danny Kruger, a Conservative MP, to consult with civil society representatives and ministers to develop proposals that would maximise the role of volunteers. His report set out a vision for a more local, less bureaucratised, less centralised society in which residents are empowered to play an active part in their neighbourhoods (Kruger, 2020).

The publication of books dealing with issues in community development has been less prolific, especially in recent years. There have been fewer discussions and critiques of community development in the United Kingdom, although those by Jacobs and Popple (1994), Popple (2000), Banks *et al.* (2003), Butcher *et al.* (2007), Henderson and Vercseg (2010), Ledwith (2020), Meade and Shaw (2021) and Chanan and Miller (2013) provide important perspectives. The collection of readings in Craig *et al.* (2011) gives a sense of the issues and debates in community development over the second half of the last century. The short guide by Gilchrist and Taylor (2022) has proved to be a useful summary of developments. The publication of *The Community Development Challenge* (DCLG, 2006) sought to strengthen community development's place on the political map.

In the European context, the drawing up of the Budapest Declaration (CEBSD/ IACD/HACD, 2004) was important in locating community development in the context of civil society. *Community Development – A European Challenge* (Brake and Deller, 2008) consists of contributions on historical movements and changes in community development. Perspectives on European community development can be found in Henderson (2005) and Henderson and Vercseg (2010).

Apart from Dominelli (2006), there have not been substantive publications on women and communities, although it is a key theme in Ledwith (2020). Perhaps driven by research undertaken on health inequalities (Wilkinson and Pickett, 2009), community development has continued to be important in the health sector (Health Empowerment Leverage Project, 2011). CHEX, which is based at the Scottish Community Development Centre, provides support and disseminates material on health issues for communities across Scotland.

From the late 1990s, neighbourhood work was drawn into the regeneration literature. The Joseph Rowntree Foundation ran three major programmes examining community-based regeneration. The publication by Taylor (2011) draws together regeneration and community development.

Church and faith-based community development work, including inter-faith work, is a significant dimension within neighbourhood work. It has been supported by a small number of publications, for example, Spratt and James (2008) and Evison (2010). The issue of community development and community care, on the other hand, has had a lower profile. Work on the issue began in the early 1990s (Armstrong and Henderson, 1992). It has been supported by a number of studies, notably Barr *et al.* (2001), and Seebohm and Gilchrist (2008).

While the issues of equalities and multiculturalism have been of major importance for community development, this has not been reflected significantly in the literature. The booklets by Gilchrist (2004, 2007) provide a framework for promoting integration and tackling inequalities.

There have been some important developments internationally (Craig and Mayo, 1995; Craig *et al.*, 2008). Two approaches to organising brought to Europe from the United States have been the Alinsky-based community organising movement (Bunyan, 2010) and asset-based community development (O'Leary *et al.*, 2011). The former has become a dynamic movement and is active in several European countries. The approach of community organising is to challenge powerholders and seek to hold them to account. Asset-based community development sees local assets – both physical and human – as the primary building blocks of sustainable community development. It is presented as an alternative to needs-based approaches to community development.

The *Community Development Journal* has continued to be a valuable source for both theory and practice, as has the International Association for Community Development. Increased links have been made in the literature between examples of practice in western and eastern/central Europe (Henderson and Vercseg, 2010) and globally (Mayo, 2005; Gaventa and Tandon, 2010; Craig *et al.*, 2011; McConnell *et al.*, 2021).

Changing context

What are the key factors and forces impacting on neighbourhoods which therefore change the ways in which neighbourhood work is practised? Here we group them under three headings: changes in experiences of neighbourhoods, the extent to which neighbourhoods have changed and the impact of external factors.

- **Changes in experiences of neighbourhoods**

For many black people and women, the neighbourhood is a place of insecurity and fear. Particularly in poor areas, extremist white groups can harass and attack black people who therefore do not experience neighbourhoods as secure, friendly places.

In recent years there has been a significant increase in the number of black and white gangs of young people roaming the streets. A shockingly high proportion of women feel threatened by the aggression and misogyny of many men. A significant number of women have also lost confidence in the police, especially following cases such as that of Sarah Everard who in 2021 was kidnapped, raped and murdered by a policeman. For many women, neighbourhoods are not necessarily safe places.

We need to note the growth of the politics of identity (Lowles and Painter, 2011): people form alliances and social movements because they share a clear identity, beliefs or values. It is a development that has become very evident in recent years especially among Black and minority ethnic communities, women and faith groups. Closely aligned to this is the phenomenon of shared interests: people come together because they have a common agenda. This could be any number of things, for example, parents of children who have a disability, elderly people who want regular social contact, people whose relatives have had COVID-19 or young people who are more likely to belong to a WhatsApp group or other social media than join a community group.

All of these represent significant changes in ways that people experience neighbourhoods and therefore have implications for neighbourhood work.

- **Extent to which neighbourhoods have changed**

It is impossible to generalise about changes in neighbourhoods. We can, however, point to some trends. One is the increased mobility of the population. People in the 2020s move in and out of neighbourhoods to a greater extent than in previous decades, according to their circumstances and choices. Greater mobility is due partly, we believe, to the increased individualism of society, a focus on the self.

There has been increased poverty with many people dependent on benefits and food banks. This has impacted severely on disadvantaged neighbourhoods. There are also growing numbers of what amount to gated communities: well-off people who want to keep disadvantaged people out.

The built environment of many neighbourhoods has changed as a result of redevelopment: new and refurbished housing, bringing in new residents. The tenure patterns of housing have changed the infrastructure of communities. Both the right to buy and the transfer of stock to social housing providers have coincided with council estates often becoming housing of last resort for the most vulnerable members of society. Accordingly, neighbourhood work on council estates faces a very different challenge compared with previous years. Social housing offers considerable opportunity for neighbourhood work. Scotland, in particular, has seen the emergence of community-based housing associations as community development organisations.

The environment has changed in other ways as well. In cities and towns, new commercial and property developments have taken over residential neighbourhoods (Minton, 2009). There have been some notable examples of inner-city residents insisting on key resources such as decent accommodation and employment for their neighbourhoods, but these have been the exception rather than the rule.

Other environmental changes have also been evident. They are as follows:

- The effects of increased car use – pollution, traffic hazards and accidents
- The dominance of large supermarkets and out-of-town shopping malls with their effect on the viability of neighbourhood shops

- The power of international corporations and banks and the influence on neighbourhoods of decisions they take
- A weakened trade union presence and reduced links between trade unions and communities.

- **The impact of external factors**

The COVID-19 pandemic has had a significant effect on people's lives and on neighbourhoods. On the one hand, during lockdown and self-isolation, individuals and families were forced to withdraw from communities. Individuals who continue to work from home will likely reinforce this. So too will the use of remote communication through the use, for example, of ZOOM. On the other hand, there was an increased sense of cohesiveness and togetherness, for example, delivering food and medicines to isolated neighbours. We shall have to see if the sense of togetherness continues in the longer term. That was the remit of the Kruger report referred to earlier. The report proposed a new Community Power Act, using deliberative democracy, participatory budgeting and citizens' assemblies. Public Health Scotland announced a new resource to support advice for community groups, organisations and volunteer networks adjusting to life with COVID-19. However, according to Groundwork, in the first six months of 2020, more than 60 per cent of community groups were forced to close or decrease their services (Groundwork, 2020).

Three other powerful external factors have been the campaigning of Black Lives Matter, the mobilisation of communities on climate change issues and Brexit. Black Lives Matter is a global political and social movement that seeks to highlight racism, discrimination and inequality experienced by black people. Black Lives Matter focuses on police violence and took off following the murder in the US of George Floyd, an African-American man, in May 2020. Black Lives Matter protests took place across the world. In the UK context, the pulling down of a statue of Edward Colston, a seventeenth-century slave trader in Bristol, was a focal point for Black Lives Matter: 'The fall of Colston marked the symbolic arrival of a new generation of young Black Britons who, along with white allies, are committed to fighting against the racism that still exists throughout much of British society' (Olusoga, 2020: 211).

Community groups have always sought to create a better local environment, particularly play areas and reduced noise, pollution and litter. They have also often united to oppose external threats such as 'fracking' (drilling for energy sources) and the destruction of the local environment as a result of new rail tracks such as HS2 from Euston to Manchester via Birmingham.

Greater public awareness of climate change and the hopes surrounding the 2021 UN climate change conference, COP 26, have increased the commitment of community groups to environmental action. One climate action group obtained a grant from its local authority to purchase a thermal imaging camera and a home energy efficiency kit box for use by residents to improve the energy use of their houses. The National Lottery has a ten-year climate action fund which will support community groups that can demonstrate what is possible when people take the lead in tackling climate change.

Brexit has led to fewer meetings of community development workers with their European counterparts. A research project commissioned by the Wales Council for Voluntary Action identified what respondents described as a 'perfect storm', whereby areas which are most in need and which have received the highest level of European

Union funding are the ones most likely to be affected by a post-Brexit downturn, leaving disadvantaged communities worse off and without the opportunities that EU funding, and the matched funding it attracted, offered.

Global politics provide the broader context, notably the contrasting presidencies of Obama, Trump and Biden (Obama's first job was as a community organiser in New York). Russia's invasion of Ukraine in February 2022 changed the global context drastically.

It is hard to make connections between the global and the local but one can identify broad lines from the one to the other: the thoughts and assumptions about global politics of people who are either already involved with their communities or who are planning to become involved.

A more tangible external factor is the extent to which planning has affected neighbourhoods, particularly Neighbourhood Plans. The idea behind them is to give communities direct power to develop a shared vision for their neighbourhood. The following is an example:

> Addingham Parish Council is the qualifying body for preparing a Neighbourhood Plan setting out how residents would like to see the village develop and improve over the next 15 years. The Plan would include matters such as protecting areas of village greenspace, supporting and encouraging local businesses, where new housing should be located, what new facilities are required, green/sustainability issues and other topics. The Neighbourhood Plan must take account of residents' views.

Our review of the changing context of neighbourhoods suggests a paradox: there are forces and influences that work against the idea of neighbourhood yet at the same time there is a continuing commitment to it. In the 1970s, Lisa Huber and Felicity McCartney were involved with the Centre for Neighbourhood Development, a voluntary agency set up to work in neighbourhoods with a population of 3,000 to 6,000 in the Greater Belfast area (Huber and McCartney, 1980). In 2022, SprengelHaus, an Intercultural Community Centre in the Wedding neighbourhood of Berlin, highlights neighbourhood development as one of the main objectives of its work (https://sprengelhaus.wedding.de). During the 50 years between these two initiatives, there have been doubts and questions raised about neighbourhood work. Austerity measures and public expenditure cuts have meant that possibilities for local authorities to employ community workers to work in neighbourhoods have declined. Yet there are new practitioners based in neighbourhoods, many of them experienced, unpaid community leaders who support local people. This continuation of classic community development has taken place alongside the emergence of the community organising movement – in 2017, the movement secured a £4.2 million contract from the Office for Civil Society to expand the number of community organisers from 6,500 to 10,000 by 2020.

It is important to note that this summary picture of community development does not apply across the whole of the United Kingdom. In Scotland, in particular, community development has remained strong. It is supported by the Scottish Centre for Community Development. Regeneration policy and legislation on community empowerment indicate a greater emphasis on communities and community assets in Scottish policy.

Both the external and internal environments of the neighbourhood have become more complex. This, together with the effects of the Internet, has meant that the significance of locality in people's lives is more difficult to identify and evaluate. Yet the neighbourhood remains a high priority for many residents. Growing numbers of people are spending more time at home and in their neighbourhood as a result of:

- early retirement, job sharing and other changes in the patterns of work, notably working from home;
- demographic changes such as the proportion of older people in the population;
- more care of disabled people including people with learning and mental health difficulties taking place in the community;
- the scarcity and cost of transport and energy, which may help to keep people more 'local' than they have been in the past;
- the impact of COVID-19 and community groups meeting on ZOOM.

The argument as to what should 'count' as economic activity has been made with increasing strength, notably by feminist social scientists and economists who question the 'invisibility' at a policy level of women's work. Child care, care of dependants, personal support, household work and involvement in local community action are mostly done by women. Thus, the reality of women's work has significant implications for neighbourhood work.

Community development

Historically the United Kingdom has played a central role in taking forward community development theory and practice from which others have learned. Is it still in a position to do this for neighbourhood work or do theory and practice now lack sufficient clarity?

Ways in which ideas of community and community practice have been incorporated within a wider spectrum of public and social policies since the early 1990s have been analysed by Butcher *et al*. (2007) and Chanan and Miller (2013). The growth of interest in 'communities of practice' (Wenger, 1998), especially through the use of e-based discussion groups, is also evidence of the extent to which interest in supporting communities has spread. It is noticeable that community development did not play a large part in these emerging themes. It is important that neighbourhood work, because it takes place at grassroots level, shares its experience and learning with wider developments.

The growth of social economy initiatives has been a positive feature of the close links that have been forged between community development and economic development. The number of social enterprises has increased significantly: cooperatives, micro-lending schemes, credit unions, community shops, housing associations, community development trusts and local exchange trading schemes. This growth area has taken place across the globe. There are many social, community and environmental schemes which do not have an economic agenda but which can be building blocks to economic development, for example, a playgroup that progresses from being mostly voluntary to a child care project with paid staff leading to a self-sustainable enterprise.

Levels of organising

We argue later why the neighbourhood is still the key level of intervention and organising for community development. It is essential, however, to relate this to other levels of organising as well as to the complexities of communities and the competing interests which exist within them. People involved in community development have had to learn how to combine the neighbourhood work approach with support for communities of interest and identity operating across much larger areas or hidden within neighbourhoods: lesbian, gay, bisexual and transgender people, people with mental health difficulties, ex-offenders and others. Support for these communities applies especially to work with women, members of minority ethnic groups and disabled people.

Information and communications technology

As we have noted already, the digital revolution has had major implications for community development. Given the power and potential of technology, innovatory use of it in neighbourhood work will undoubtedly continue. We need to note, however, that in 2020 more than 6 per cent of adults in the United Kingdom had never used the Internet. It is the old, poor and unemployed who are least likely to use it. Online and mobile technologies increase the range of possibilities for people to connect with others. The technologies help to generate network capital. Facebook, Twitter, local digital media and other options have opened up a new sphere for communication and the building of relationships and also for organising, critiquing and protesting.

Online tools and resources are being used increasingly to support neighbourhood work practice. For example, in Scotland, where community engagement is part of the Scottish Executive's mainstream policy, Visioning Outcomes in Community Engagement (VOiCE) provides online access for professionals to analyse, plan, conduct and evaluate engagement (www.voicesscotland.org.uk). Learning, Evaluation and Planning (LEAP) offers a similar function for planning and evaluating community initiatives (www.planandevaluate.com).

Governance and community development

In recent years there has been increased commitment to citizen action and participation. Citizens' juries and participatory budgeting are two examples. This has coincided with continuing evidence of the disaffection of electors with formal democratic processes. Neighbourhood work has a key role to play in supporting active citizenship (Mayo and Annette, 2010). This is particularly important because most local authorities are too large to connect meaningfully with local people. They are also dominated by central government controls. Residents of the inner-city neighbourhoods may be reluctant to vote in elections but they can be mobilised around local issues: participatory democracy can flourish alongside representative democracy (Forbrig, 2011).

Modernising community development

Research undertaken in the early 1990s provided evidence for the existence of the community sector as being distinct from, albeit linked to, the voluntary sector (Chanan, 1997). Essentially, the community sector consists of the aggregate of small voluntary organisations, community groups and informal networks. It contrasts with the professionalised voluntary sector. From the mid-1990s onwards, the term 'community sector' became an accepted part of policy discussions relating both to community development and the commitment of regeneration programmes, planning and housing to involving communities. Recognition of the role and value of a distinct community sector has made a significant additional contribution to arguments put forward for community development. Research by the Third Sector Research Centre provided evidence for the existence of community groups and organisations that exist 'below the radar' at local level or in communities of interest: groups and organisations, which are not easily identifiable and which come and go but nevertheless have considerable significance for communities (McCabe and Phillmore, 2010).

Given the need to modernise community development, we should expect to find a diverse range of practice examples. The following is from Crossroads, a longstanding community organisation in Glasgow:

> Crossroads has employed community workers for all its 50+ years but the model of practice has evolved. Our community development programme in Gorbals works with individuals and groups to identify and develop existing strengths and assets and create stronger community connections resulting in new, positive actions and experiences for people. . . . Our workers harness people's strengths to establish activities they want, creating supportive relationships. Through their active involvement, learning and sharing new skills, and supporting each other, people also build confidence and self-esteem.
>
> (Stuart Hashagen, personal communication)

The example indicates the extent to which the process of neighbourhood work as set out in this book has been developed in different ways.

Until the government introduced major public expenditure cuts in 2011, one could have been optimistic that local authorities would continue to play a key role in supporting community development. This was because government policies on partnership working and localism looked to local authorities to coordinate and implement these ideas. Now one is less sanguine that they are in a position to do this. Neighbourhood work will need to search out other resources to provide support. It could, for example, connect with co-production models. Co-production is focused on new ways of delivering public services by building relationships between service providers, service users and wider community resources. The New Economics Foundation aims to encourage agencies to work with community members to co-design and co-deliver outcomes that are meaningful and sustainable.

Over the last 20 years, governments and funders have insisted that organisations specify clear outcomes and outputs. This has meant that community development has had to improve its approach to planning and evaluation. It is no longer possible for organisations to have open-ended community development programmes. In Chapter 2, we show how evaluation models for neighbourhood work can provide a robust response to critics who argue that neighbourhood work is a too general and unclear intervention to keep pace with the planning and evaluation requirements of modernisation.

Key concepts

It has been a paradox of community development in the United Kingdom that its practitioners, writers and trainers have done little to develop ideas about the neighbourhood – a paradox because it has been neighbourhood work that has predominantly characterised community practice. Most of the analysis and discussion of neighbourhood work have centred on community engagement. This has prioritised the vertical relationships between community groups and resource holders and decision makers, and on the means by which such groups can obtain the resources they need as well as influence policy and planning decisions. This concern with communities taking action has rarely been matched by an interest in community interaction. Social development has not kept pace with economic and physical regeneration but a debate about building community resilience and community assets has emerged. That is why the concept of social capital that we summarise in the following section has so much relevance to neighbourhood work. Yet there remains a poverty of theorising about networks and linkages, roles and relationships, and the extent and quality of people's interactions. The work of Alison Gilchrist on networking as an essential component of community development is a welcome contribution (Gilchrist, 2019).

With the exception of the Community Development Projects (1968–77), social policy in the United Kingdom has had a *laisser-faire* attitude to the development of communities. Even within the more recent regeneration programmes, the neighbourhood has been seen as the zone or framework within which other social systems operate; rarely has the neighbourhood been seen as a unit in its own right, as an important element of social structure about which we should ask evaluative questions on its functioning and condition – and how it can be supported. What we particularly lack is a generic theory of the neighbourhood and neighbourhood work. By this we mean a theory that makes sense to, and is usable by, a whole range of practitioners engaged in neighbourhood life.

Social capital

Research carried out by Robert Putnam, first in Italy and then in the United States, showed the relationship between social processes and community infrastructure and economic development. Social capital refers both to networks and trust between people and to the relationship between people and institutions. It can be highly significant in building strong communities, combating social exclusion and providing an essential basis for long-term economic development. Putnam shows that very poor people living in inner-city areas who have a relatively small number of intense family and neighbourhood gang ties and loyalties are trapped in their poverty, whereas those who have a wider network of more dispersed contacts do better (Putnam, 2000). Trust and cooperation are the crucial elements of social capital. Woolcock (2001), also published in Gilchrist (2019), argues that each of the following kinds of social capital is necessary for strong and sustainable communities:

- *Bonding*. Based on enduring, multi-faceted relationships between similar people with strong mutual commitments such as among friends, family and other close-knit groups;
- *Bridging*. Formed from the connections between people who have less in common, but may have an overlapping interest, for example, between neighbours, colleagues, or between different groups within a community; and
- *Linking*. Derived from the links between people or organisations beyond peer boundaries, cutting across status and similarity and enabling people to exert influence and reach resources outside their normal circles.

The concept of social capital is used in a wide variety of community development settings. Ways in which it connects with neighbourhood work include the following:

- It is only possible to do neighbourhood work if local people are motivated to give their time and energy voluntarily. It is very difficult to work effectively when there is a high level of disaffection, distrust and a lack of cooperation. In other words, for neighbourhood work to succeed there has to be a focus on building hope and trust and there must be potential for cooperation.
- Neighbourhood work sets out to build upon weak or perhaps neglected aspects of social capital: while a lot of work will be undertaken with particular individuals, its main interest is in bringing people together into informal groups and then more formal organisations. The words 'enable', 'facilitate' and 'encourage' constantly recur in neighbourhood work because it is always looking for ways of encouraging people to plan and act together, thus developing collective rather than individual action. It is this notion to which phrases such as 'self-help' and 'community action' refer.
- Yet neighbourhood work depends on there being individuals who can help to explain what it is that an initiative is aiming to achieve and who can convince neighbours and others that it is worthwhile giving the initiative a chance. People, in short, who are key members and connectors of local informal networks.
- Practitioners have to be highly active and present within communities – it is in this way that they build up people's commitment and willingness to join an organisation. However, they also have to operate within and between the organisations and institutions whose policies and programmes impact powerfully on communities. Practitioners have to build up their own networks so that they can both look into and be involved with a neighbourhood and look outward, linking with the local authority, health and other agencies. It can be seen how these dimensions relate to the concept of social capital.
- Neighbourhood work can lead to engagement by local people with powerholders and different forms of governance. Marilyn Taylor describes how communities, where there has been capacity building, can engage with other players to create community change (Taylor, 2011).

Civil society

The emergence of civil society as a concept which, across the globe, underpins expressions of popular movements and community action has been remarkable. Its meaning may be contested but the idea at its core is universal. It was key to the revolutions in eastern and central Europe at the end of the 1980s. It is about the determination of ordinary people to organise themselves in ways that either bring them into dialogue with the state or that lead them to challenge or confront the state.

In the UK context, the concept has been linked to ideas of active citizenship and empowerment. Like the term community development, the concept of civil society is used elastically and is adopted across a broad political spectrum. It is of central importance in understanding and explaining community development. Henderson and Vercseg put forward five ways in which community development can help communities be part of civil society: challenging, defending, maintaining, recognising and strengthening civil society (Henderson and Vercseg, 2010: 23–27).

Social inclusion

The purpose of social inclusion strategies is to tackle inequalities and generate a greater sense of social cohesion. The term social inclusion is preferred by many people to that of social exclusion because the former is more positive; its use has moved a long way from being associated only with anti-poverty work. It embraces the idea of participation. A determination to counter assumptions that poor people lack the motivation and skills to do things for themselves is central to community development thinking. The concept of social inclusion is especially important for black and minority ethnic people in their struggles against racism and their right to participate as full members of society through processes of equal access and integration.

A more pragmatic reason for seeing social inclusion as a key underpinning idea in neighbourhood work is the reality that anti-poverty programmes will not succeed unless communities are mobilised to become stronger. In this sense, anti-poverty measures and participation are two sides of the same coin. Neighbourhood work can initiate and support schemes that provide specific benefits and services, for example:

- food cooperatives to enable people to buy good quality food at affordable prices;
- credit unions to help people save and borrow money at low cost;
- community and social enterprises which employ local people and provide services for communities.

Building community capacity

The term 'capacity building' has become inseparable from the policy and practice of regeneration. It is used to apply both to individuals and to groups. Emphasis is given to its systematic approach towards helping residents play a major part in the regeneration of their neighbourhood. It is also used with other stakeholders to help them work effectively with communities. This is a key argument developed by the Scottish Community Development Centre: it is not just the people who experience the need that we should think about but also the people who can support activity to bring about change, those who might work in partnership with them and equally those who might actively resist attempts to achieve change.

Capacity building has a focus on training: 'activities, resources and support that strengthen the skills, abilities and confidence of people and community groups to take effective action and leading roles in the development of communities' (Skinner, 2006: 4). There is a danger that capacity building can be used as an instrumental term, part of the agenda of economic development organisations rather than a response to the learning needs of residents who want to have the understanding and confidence to participate on equal terms.

The educative strand of neighbourhood work is vital: the processes of learning and change, usually experiential and informal, which can take place as part of community action and activities. Both training courses and occupational standards for community development need to ensure that this dimension of neighbourhood work remains central. At the same time it is important to provide opportunities for exploring alternative approaches to working with communities other than those that appear to be dominant. This perspective reflects the influence of Paulo Freire on adult education and community development, especially his argument that critical dialogue and reflection on action, as well as explicit value sets, are essential for effective and sustainable action (Freire, 1972).

Towards community capability

The idea of building community capacity links to good practice in neighbourhood work. It is concerned with the development of confidence and skills of local people, the strengthening of local organisations, and the development of open and inclusive networks. It also addresses the issues of efficiency and resilience of community groups and organisations. There is widespread recognition that all stakeholders need to develop the capacity to work with each other.

We think that an idea which is closely akin to that of capacity building is the idea of 'community capability'. It speaks to the need for a generic theory of the neighbourhood and neighbourhood work referred to at the beginning of this section on key concepts. It does not, however, have the functional connotation of capacity building, and it addresses the need to build relationships within neighbourhoods.

The idea of community capability is taken from the research of Wallman (1982), Schoenberg (1979) and Schoenberg and Rosenbaum (1980), who explored the concept of the viability of local communities and the ways in which residents pursue their livelihoods. Behind these meanings of community capability, there lies a wider general notion, defined by Schoenberg in the following way:

> Viable neighbourhoods are differentiated by the fact that these are neighbourhoods in which residents can control the local social order. Residents in such neighbourhoods set the goals for collective life, and they have the ability to implement programmes to accomplish these goals.
>
> (Schoenberg, 1979: 69)

Following, but building upon Schoenberg's work, we would say that a neighbourhood achieves this kind of capability if it can:

- establish mechanisms to negotiate and implement shared agreements or contracts about public roles and responsibilities. These would vary from neighbourhood to neighbourhood but would certainly include agreements about personal safety, the identification of strangers, the maintenance of common property, the disposal of rubbish and the behaviour of children;
- set up both formal and informal organisations in the locality which provide for communication, the emergence of leadership, the learning of skills, and the ability to define, and take action upon, the various interests of the neighbourhood to those outside it;
- make inputs – through representation, advocacy and campaigning – on policy and political decision-making that affects the neighbourhood;
- maintain linkages to public and private resource holders;
- establish consultation, negotiation and exchange mechanisms, formal and informal, through which dialogue and conflict resolution are created between different interests, needs and groups in the neighbourhood.

In all these functions it is important to ensure that all groups and interests have opportunities to be included and involved, especially minorities and those protected under equalities legislation.

In most deprived neighbourhoods these kinds of mechanisms and organisation will not be created or sustained without the support and intervention of neighbourhood work practitioners and the provision of basic administrative and servicing resources. Key to the approach of practitioners will be dealing with tensions and unequal power dynamics and looking for opportunities for integration, cross-cultural learning and celebration.

The challenge faced by professionals in fields such as housing, health, regeneration and education is to realise that they must seek not just to deliver services to meet people's needs but also to do so in ways that enhance people's autonomy, self-esteem and their ability to work together to solve common problems. This is at the heart of the idea of public service reform, co-production and prevention. Pressures to involve voluntary organisations and community groups in the delivery of services underscore the importance of this point. At the heart of the development of capable communities is the understanding that the way in which professionals carry out their professional role – that is, the neighbourhood-sensitive way in which they carry it out – is as important as meeting the needs of individuals.

Networking

Neighbourhood work practitioners need to see themselves as helping to develop communities into capable social systems, rather than agents of particular community or identity groups with a specific but limited task. Clearly, the creation and support of such action groups are essential to collective problem-solving but they need to be seen as a crucial part of the development of a strong, interacting community. Neighbourhood workers, other practitioners and policy-makers should seek to develop their understanding and skills in promoting horizontal integration at the locality level. Their job is not only to help local people establish the kinds of organisations and networks necessary for community capability but also to support people's participation in them, to make them effective, to raise the issue of membership in groups, to promote inclusion and tackle barriers to participation, to challenge prejudice and discrimination and to facilitate access and choice. Introducing and sustaining imaginative ways of disseminating information and communicating is a necessary part of this work.

Neighbourhood work is about putting people in touch with one another, promoting their membership in groups and building networks of contacts and relationships both within and beyond the neighbourhood. It seeks to develop people's sense of power and significance in acts of association with others that may also achieve some improvement in their social and material well-being. The outcomes of neighbourhood work that are possible, such as increased community cohesion and reduction in the fear of crime, can be seen to be an essential part of governance. That is why it is important to evaluate the short-term and long-term effects of neighbourhood work.

Neighbourhood work is concerned with political, organisational and personal development. At its best, it combines both organisational and individual changes. At its most potent, it is concerned not simply with the system or individual but also with *role*: it is an intervention that helps people to develop and expand the roles which they have been accustomed to taking – or not taking – in life, exercising their rights as citizens and supporting them to take on responsibilities as community members. It works on the interface between private troubles and public issues, and between the individual and the collective, demonstrating that working in this way can be effective in bringing about change. This is why the training and education dimensions are so important. So too is time for reflection and planning.

The relational aspect of neighbourhood renewal means the building of trust and solidarity between people who, as residents, often have different priorities and who may have different roles and responsibilities with other stakeholders. In the act of bringing people together, neighbourhood work practitioners are performing an essential role. They have the much-needed skill of helping people associate with one another in a society where many of the forces at work separate and atomise them. As workers put people in touch with one another, neighbourhood work gives priority to those in greatest need, and it is able to do this without stigmatising them.

Seeing neighbourhood work as a process

We have found it valuable to see neighbourhood work as a process of development. The usefulness of a process account is to make explicit the variety of tasks that practitioners carry out in their work with neighbourhood groups. The act of establishing process provides a way of *identifying, distinguishing, ordering* and *categorising* the activities of the neighbourhood worker.

Identifying the elements of practice is of help in alerting the practitioner to what needs to be done in his or her work and how it should be carried out. In particular, the worker may see the varying needs of groups at different stages of the process, and this in turn may be suggestive of the different roles, skills and knowledge likely to be required of the worker.

Distinguishing the different aspects of neighbourhood work may help those responsible for training, support, management and supervision better to identify the ways in which they can contribute to the skill development of students and practitioners.

The *ordering* of the elements of practice turns our attention to the timing, sequencing and inter-relatedness of the worker's interventions. Specifically, the act of sorting the parts of the work underlines the need for planning the worker's activities. For example, success in carrying out the end phase of neighbourhood work is contingent upon decisions the practitioner makes, or fails to make, at the beginning of the intervention. Attempts at evaluation may be frustrated because of inattention in the early phases to setting up appropriate recording procedures. The kind of withdrawal a worker makes from a group may be determined by the kind of role established with the group since the first contact with them.

The *categorising* of neighbourhood work practice not only imposes 'order' on the various activities that comprise the worker's day-to-day practice but also facilitates the identification of similarities in the work of different practitioners engaged with groups from different neighbourhoods pursuing a range of issues. The ability to categorise our work, and to generalise from it, is an important step towards the strengthening of practice theory in neighbourhood work.

A process view of neighbourhood work also points to the dynamic elements of our interventions. Through process accounts we may better understand the *purposeful* nature of the work. The fact that the interventions of practitioners have intentionality and direction is important to grasp because in the actual doing of neighbourhood work, practitioners often feel caught in a turbulent environment of community activities, politics and dynamics, with little immediate sense of where their work is leading them or the group with whom they work.

Of course, the working situation for the practitioner often is unpredictable and confusing. The ability to conceive of one's activity at any point as part of an ongoing process provides not only sense and direction but also the opportunity to disengage and stand back from action. We suggest that the activity of 'taking stock' is an important element in the process of neighbourhood work.

We present here our account of the process of neighbourhood work that provides the main structure for this book. Our treatment of some of the initial stages of the process reflects its urban origin and readers interested, for example, in rural, suburban or new town environments must adapt and add to our discussion in order to increase its relevance to these situations. Nevertheless, we believe that our discussion of ideas and principles is relevant to a variety of community and professional contexts. Our nine-stage process of neighbourhood work is as follows:

- Entering the neighbourhood
- Getting to know the neighbourhood
- What next? Needs, goals and roles
- Making contacts and bringing people together
- Forming and building organisations
- Helping to clarify goals and priorities
- Keeping the organisation going
- Dealing with friends and enemies
- Leavings and endings

A few points about this process: it does not portray the phases through which a group, or a neighbourhood, moves, though there is some discussion of group development and process in Chapter 9. Our process defines the major areas of work that any worker will be engaged in if she sees some neighbourhood action through from beginning to end. This is not to say that each piece of neighbourhood work will necessarily and always involve the practitioner in these major tasks; we believe that every practitioner in each piece of neighbourhood work will be involved in some of these phases and tasks, and that our process defines the major areas of work that any worker will be engaged in if he or she sees some neighbourhood action through from beginning to end.

There are clearly a good many interconnections between each of the stages in the process. In practice, the stages do not represent discrete categories of tasks, skills and knowledge. The activities of each stage prepare for, and feed into, the subsequent stages, and there is, and ought to be, feedback from each stage to the worker about what has been achieved in preceding stages. Some of the stages continue as ongoing tasks for the practitioner. For example, the activities of data collection and making contacts are ever-present responsibilities for the worker, and are usually improved both qualitatively and quantitatively by a worker's tasks in stages of the process that are, in our account, subsequent to them. In brief, the process is not a simple sequential or linear one; most of the stages overlap and interact with one or some of the others.

We believe that our account of the process of neighbourhood work provides a basic kit of terms, ideas and frameworks. As with most kits, it is our hope that readers will play around with it, adding and subtracting bits, in order to produce something that is suited to their needs and interests. A kit, after all, is only as good as the shapes and functions to which its users can put it.

There is a danger that too much will be expected of the neighbourhood work process. The reader will have noted that – for reasons of space – we have given only slight attention to some skill areas for neighbourhood work (including undertaking a community profile, recording and supervision). It is essential both that the practitioners obtain such knowledge and skill and remain aware of the need to update it. It is for this reason that we have a chapter on evaluation.

Neighbourhood work has to provoke energy, interest and sense of excitement. Much of its strength comes from its search for more effective and meaningful methods, tactics and strategies. Without this, it risks becoming arid and moribund.

By itself the process account is insufficient for practising neighbourhood work. Values, ideology and creativity constitute the lifeblood of organising and action at local level. They require that anger, passion, caring, determination and a host of other emotions and expressions of commitments be part of the daily vocabulary of practitioners. The process model has to lie alongside these, not dominate them. Furthermore, writing practice theory for neighbourhood work has to be combined with an explicit values framework such as that provided by the International Association for Community Development. This emphasises the promotion of participative democracy, sustainable development, rights, economic opportunity, equality and social justice (www.iacdglobal.org/about).

A workbook

We have worked on the assumption that readers will want to adapt the model set out in this book, amending and adding to it according to their experience and their ideas about how practice should develop. It may be, for example, that people will want to expand those parts which deal with the day-to-day work with community groups and their management. The balance of the material is weighted more towards planning an intervention, making contact and forming groups. We would encourage people to wrestle with the book in that way. It is also essential to ensure that learning and skills are part of practice; they are central to the material in this publication and how we suggest it is used.

Neighbourhood workers are often tempted to tackle every situation which they encounter, and many times they are under pressure to do so. Training, supervision and reflection seek to counter this tendency. Neighbourhood practitioners may form part of a team of professionals, but the isolated nature of their work can be a problem. They may lack the close support of colleagues working on the same task. If they want that kind of support, they usually have to make a point of deliberately acquiring it from co-workers who have different tasks. Peer supervision is one possibility:

> I once had a formal arrangement with another neighbourhood worker in which we would take it in turns to talk about our practice and be 'supervised' – one month as supervisor, next month as supervisee. No money changed hands. It worked very well.
>
> (Gilchrist, A., personal communication)

Or neighbourhood workers can seek the support they need from key members of community groups with whom they are working. This can be combined with them accessing funds from within their organisation to enable them to pay for a series of meetings with a consultant. This person can help them to understand the policy and organisational context in which they are working. Part of the work of 'situating oneself', which we look at in Chapter 3, involves understanding, adjusting to and influencing this policy context.

These different forms of support and development can help the practitioner to constantly consider the question 'why?' Why are you planning to carry out a survey? Why are you attending every meeting of such and such a group? The legitimacy of making such challenges lies in the belief that standing back from the action, examining a piece of work critically with the help of someone who is to an extent outside it, will result in more thoughtful and therefore more effective work being accomplished.

Neighbourhood workers can experience isolation because of the nature of the work they do. They appear to have roving agendas, moving between contrasting scenarios, for example, a meeting with the chairperson of a trust, booking a hall for a community group's jumble sale, time on websites to collect information on a neighbourhood, helping a group carry out a survey, an interview with a planning officer about a possible play area. Neighbourhood workers often have to handle such situations within a short time period, and they are therefore always working with different audiences and constituencies. The role requires considerable flexibility and versatility and the ability to be comfortable working across and between boundaries. This is a theme we shall return to; it makes an interesting contrast to the 'public' nature of the worker's job carried out at meetings, conferences and social events. Here we draw attention to the 'loner' position into which a worker can be forced. Finding support from others and working within a clear practice framework are priorities for a worker.

In Chapter 3, we take the reader through the main phases of the process. A worker will draw upon the same knowledge and skills for different parts of the process, and we try to indicate this. The occasional reappearance of material in chapters, or reference to skills already identified, is therefore not accidental.

We often wondered when writing this book whether it might appear too detailed and comprehensive. There is a danger that we elaborate the process of neighbourhood work so much as to discourage anyone from embarking on it. Perhaps we have provided prescriptions which no one will feel they have the skills, energy and time to follow in practice. We must stress, therefore, that what we have written should be used more as a source of ideas on particular points rather than be read through at one sitting. For example, trainers and students may read a chapter as a preparation for discussing specific skills, and this might be followed by a seminar on issues that have emerged from the chapter and discussion. In the acknowledgements at the beginning of the book, we refer to the workshops on neighbourhood work skills that we ran and we think that the book can be used in training courses of that kind – identifying and practising skills in a safe learning environment – and these can dovetail with other educational methods.

References

Armstrong, J. and Henderson, P. (1992) 'Putting the community into community care', *Community Development Journal*, 27, 2: 189–92.

Banks, S., Butcher, H., Henderson, P. and Robertson, J. (eds) (2003) *Managing community practice; principles, policies and programmes*, Bristol: The Policy Press.

Barr, A. (1996) *Practising community development. Experience in Strathclyde*, London: CDF Publications.

Barr, A., Stenhouse, C. and Henderson, P. (2001) *Caring communities. A challenge for social inclusion*, York: York Publishing Services.

Brake, R. and Deller, U. (eds) (2008) *Community development – A European challenge*, Opladen and Farmington Hills: Barbara Budrich Publishers.

Bunyan, P. (2010) 'Broad-based organising in the UK: reasserting the centrality of political activity in community development', *Community Development Journal*, 45, 1: 111–27.

Butcher, H., Banks, S., Henderson, P. with Robertson, J. (2007) *Critical community practice*, Bristol: The Policy Press.

CEBSD/IACD/HACD (Combined European Bureau for Social Development/International Association for Community Development/Hungarian Association for Community Development) (2004) *The Budapest declaration. Building European civil society through community development*. Online. Available HTTP: <www.cebsd.org> (accessed 10 January 2012).

Chanan, G. (1997) *Active citizenship and community involvement*, Dublin: European Foundation for the Improvement of Living and Working Conditions.

Chanan, G. and Miller, C. (2013) *Rethinking community practice: developing transformative neighbourhoods*, Bristol: The Policy Press.

Craig, G. and Mayo, M. (1995) *Community empowerment. A reader in participation and development*, London: Zed Books.

Craig, G., Mayo, M., Popple, K., Shaw, M. and Taylor, M. (2011) *The community development reader: History, themes and issues*, Bristol: The Policy Press.

Craig, G., Popple, K. and Shaw, M. (2008) *Community development in theory and practice: An international reader*, Nottingham: Spokesman.

Department for Communities and Local Government (DCLG). (2002) *The learning curve – developing skills and knowledge for neighbourhood renewal*, London: DCLG.

Department for Communities and Local Government (DCLG). (2006) *The community development challenge*, London: DCLG.

Derounian, J. G. (1998) *Effective working with rural communities*, Chichester: Packard Publishing Ltd.

Dominelli, L. (2006) *Women and collective action* (2nd edn), Bristol: The Policy Press.

Egan. (2004) *The Egan review: skills for sustainable communities*, London: Communities and Local Government.

Evison, I. (2010) *Faith matters. Case studies from the faith in action fund*, London: CDF.

Forbrig, ed. (2011) *Learning for local democracy. A study of local citizen participation in Europe*, CALLDE. Online. Available HTTP: <www.ceen.net> (accessed 19 March 2012).

Francis, D. and Henderson, P. (1992) *Working with rural communities*, Basingstoke: Macmillan.

Freire, P. (1972) *Pedagogy of the oppressed*, Harmondsworth: Penguin.

Gaventa, J. and Tandon, R. (eds) (2010) *Globalising citizens: new dynamics of inclusion and exclusion*, London: Zed Books.

Gilchrist, A. (2004) *Community development and community cohesion: bridges or barricades?* London: CDF.

Gilchrist, A. (2007) *Equalities and communities: challenge, choice and change*, London: CDF.

Gilchrist, A. (2019) *The well-connected community: a networking approach to community development* (3rd edn), Bristol: The Policy Press.

Gilchrist, A. and Taylor, M. (2022) *The short guide to community development* (3rd edn), Bristol: The Policy Press.

Groundwork (2020) Community groups in a crisis. Insights from the first six months of the Covid-19 pandemic. <www.groundwork.org.uk> (accessed 24 April 2022).

Hawtin, M. and Percy-Smith, J. (2007) *Community profiling. A practical guide* (2nd edn), Maidenhead: Open University Press.

Huber, L. and McCartney, F. (1980) 'Community work in Belfast: A neighbourhood approach', in P. Henderson, D. N. Jones and D. N. Thomas (eds.) *The boundaries of change in community work*, London: George Allen and Unwin.

Health Empowerment Leverage Project. (2011) *Empowering communities for health: business case and practice framework*. Online. Available HTTP: <www.healthempowermentgroup. org.uk> (accessed 19 February 2012).

Henderson, P. (2005) *Including the excluded*, Bristol: The Policy Press.

Henderson, P. and Vercseg, I. (2010) *Community development and civil society*, Bristol: The Policy Press.

Jacobs, S. and Popple, K. (1994) *Community work in the 1990s*, Nottingham: Spokesman.

Kruger, D. (2020) *Levelling up our communities: proposals for a new social covenant*, London: Dept. for Digital, Culture, Media & Sport.

Ledwith, M. (2020) *Community development. A critical approach* (3rd edn), Bristol: The Policy Press.

Lowles, N. and Painter, A. (2011) *Fear and HOPE. The new politics of identity*, London: Searchlight Educational Trust.

Mayo, M. (2005) *Global citizens. Social movements and the challenge of globalisation*, London: Zed Books.

Mayo, M. and Annette, J. (2010) *Taking part? Active learning for active citizenship and beyond*, Leicester: National Institute of Adult Continuing Education (England and Wales).

McCabe, A. and Phillmore, J. (eds) (2010) *Below the radar in a big society? Reflections on community engagement, empowerment and social action in a changing context*, Third Sector Research Centre (University of Birmingham), working paper 51. Online. Available HTTP: <www.trrc.ac.uk> (accessed 21 February 2012).

McConnell, C., Muia, D. and Clarke, A. (eds) (2021) *International community development practice – community development research and practice series*, New York, NY: IACD/Taylor & Francis.

Meade, R. and Shaw, M. (eds) (2021) *Arts, culture and community development (rethinking community development)*, Bristol: The Policy Press.

Minton, A. (2009) *Ground control. Fear and happiness in the twenty-first century city*, London: Penguin Books.

New Economics Foundation. (1998) *Participation works!* London: NEF.

O'Leary, T., Burkett, I. and Braithwaite, K. (2011) *Appreciating assets*, Dunfermline: Carnegie UK Trust/International Association for Community Development. Online. Available HTTP: <www.iacdglobal.org> (accessed 29 February 2012).

Olusoga, D. (2020). *Black and British: A forgotten history*, London: Picador Books.

Pitchford, M. with Henderson, P. (2008) *Making spaces for community development*, London: CDF.

Popple, K. (2000) *Analysing community work. Its theory and practice* (2nd edn), Buckingham: Open University Press.

Putnam, R. (2000) *Bowling alone. The collapse and revival of American community*, New York: Simon & Schuster.

Richardson, L. (2008) *DIY community action. Neighbourhood problems and community self-help*, Bristol: The Policy Press.

Schoenberg, S. P. (1979) 'Criteria for the evaluation of neighbourhood viability in working-class and low income areas in core cities', *Social Problems*, 27, 1.

Schoenberg, S. P. and Rosenbaum, P. L. (1980) *Neighbourhoods that work: sources for viability in the inner city*, New Brunswick, NJ: Rutgers University Press.

Seebohm, P. and Gilchrist, A. (2008) *Connect and include. An exploratory study of community development and mental health*, London: National Social Inclusion Programme in association with CDF.

Skinner, S. (2006) *Strengthening communities. A guide to capacity building for communities and the public sector*, London: CDF.

Smith, M. (1994) *Local education*, Buckingham: Open University Press.

Spratt, E. and James, M. (2008) *Faith, cohesion and community development* (2nd edn), London: CDF.

Taylor, M. (2011) *Public policy in the community* (2nd edn), Basingstoke: Palgrave Macmillan.

Twelvetrees, A. (2008) *Community work* (4th edn), Basingstoke: Palgrave Macmillan.

Wallman, S. (1982) *Living in south London*, London: Gower.

Wenger, E. (1998) *Communities of practice: learning, meaning and identity*, Cambridge: Cambridge University Press.

Wilkinson, R. and Pickett, K. (2009) *The spirit level*, London: Penguin Books.

Wilson, M. and Wilde, P. (2001) *Building practitioner strengths*, London: CDF.

Woolcock, M. (2001) 'The place of social capital in understanding social and economic outcomes', *ISUMA Canadian Journal of Policy Research*, 2, 1: 11–17.

2   Thinking about evaluation

Evaluation is often associated with endings in neighbourhood work. We suggest, however, that the worker begins thinking about evaluation as something which is ongoing and which should be thought about at the very start of working in a neighbourhood. That is why we place the chapter here, and not at the end of the book.

There has been general recognition that evaluation is essential in neighbourhood work. It can be carried out by a public body, a voluntary organisation or a community group, and be funded as a grant, a contract or a service. However it is funded and organised, evaluation is the main way of establishing whether

- a project provides value for money;
- it is achieving the change that is sought or;
- demonstrating that new ideas or proposals are valid.

Most people now accept evaluation as a necessary, if not always welcome, process, as a way of showing that the funds that are available for community development are providing benefits, and that these benefits are clear and identifiable. Moreover, good practice demands a degree of curiosity to understand the effects of things that were done, and the possibility of considering whether things would have been different had other actions taken place. Such curiosity is important in reaching a better understanding of practice. It could be argued that thinking about evaluation is the key to good practice in planning. Perhaps even more important in times of economic stringency is the need to demonstrate that investment in neighbourhood work is cost-effective – in terms of either added value or reduced costs elsewhere.

It is essential to be clear about what neighbourhood work can be expected to do – and what may be beyond its powers. For example, it may be advocated as a means of improving community health, increasing employability or combatting poverty. While neighbourhood work may well help create the conditions in which such ambitions may be realised, it does not in itself necessarily lead to these outcomes. We therefore need to understand how neighbourhood work can build the strengths and effectiveness of local groups and organisations, as well as their ability to bring about needed change in their areas.

DOI: 10.4324/9781003310006-2

Why evaluate?

A useful starting point is to recognise that planning and evaluation are two sides of the same coin – it is difficult to do one without having thought about the other. If you give some thought to what it is that you – and the communities you work with – would like to have in place after a given period of time, then you will have a good starting point to consider how you might seek to get to that point. Equally, you would need to consider how you would know whether your plans had had the anticipated effect, and how you might develop your practice from this knowledge.

As well as being basic good practice, evaluation is increasingly required by agencies and funders of neighbourhood work; indeed, rare is the project or activity that does not require some form of evaluation. The challenge for neighbourhood work practice is whether the terms of the evaluation as set out by the sponsoring agency are consistent with the practice and its intended outcomes. The more that these terms and outcomes are negotiated and agreed, the more useful evaluation will be.

Government bodies and other funders increasingly require information on the relationship between action and effect. In many ways this places the responsibility for good quality evaluation with any practitioner or agency that seeks to secure future funding. Thus the demand for evaluation from sponsors is now equalled by the recognition of many in the field that it is also in their best interest to conduct thorough evaluation, to record learning and to base further planning on what has been learned.

Engaging with communities has been identified as adding value to the 'normal' delivery of public services because they are more likely to respond to the needs and preferences of the recipients, and more likely to complement community activities. For example, Audit Scotland, the body in Scotland that scrutinises how public money is spent, tries to assess how well an organisation demonstrates a commitment to engaging with communities. It asks questions on leadership, culture and capacity building.

As well as being important to funders and sponsors, neighbourhood workers themselves can find that paying attention to evaluation can be a good way to generate the insights that are the basis of developing practice competence, as well as confidence in one's practice. A reflective practitioner will value the understanding gained from asking critical questions about what happens, how and why it happens, and what his or her role is. Such learning can be invaluable the next time around, and this applies as much to a community group or project as to a worker.

When shared with local people, evaluation can become more powerful still. There are interesting examples of projects inviting the neighbourhood with which they are working to define the outcomes and measures of success that they would wish to use or see. Such an approach provides a focus for both the worker and the neighbourhood. It also holds people to account and emphasises the importance of evaluation so that all those who are interested will understand what happened, what didn't, and why.

As well as encouraging a dialogue with local people about their issues and ambitions, preparing for evaluation also provides a good opportunity to explain what the neighbourhood work role involves. This can make the worker more accountable to the community, thereby achieving greater legitimacy and confidence.

A robust approach to evaluation, combined with conveying clear messages as to what neighbourhood work is – and is not – about, would help address criticisms that it is a well-meaning but woolly intervention. Good evaluation and good planning are based on clarity of purpose and a clear sense of direction, negotiated as far as possible with the neighbourhoods in question. Such clarity should include:

- an indication of the outcomes that are sought and why they would be expected to have a beneficial impact;
- a statement of the methods to be adopted to achieve the outcomes intended;
- an understanding of the roles and tasks involved.

If such practices could be more widely adopted, the case for greater investment in neighbourhood work would be much stronger. There would be clearer evidence to demonstrate its value and purpose, and indeed its cost-effectiveness. In a climate of financial stringency this is vital: there is good evidence that investing in communities can both reduce costs to the public purse and enhance benefits to the community. This is known as the social return on investment. The Christie Commission reviewed public services in Scotland and made the case for services to be built around communities and their needs (Christie, 2011). In England, the Health Empowerment Leverage Project explores the business case for the use of community development in health (Health Empowerment Leverage Project, 2011).

What are the issues?

If a considered approach to evaluation has the advantages described earlier, why is it seen as problematic or burdensome? There are several reasons. The most immediate response from practitioners is often that it takes up too much time, that it is not really necessary, and that in a busy and demanding occupation it is better to prioritise work with people and groups. But if you don't spend time evaluating (and developing your skills for doing so) then your practice may suffer or fail to progress. Evaluation is a recognised competency in community work, an essential skill for practice and accountability.

Practitioners might also see evaluation as imposed from above, something the practitioner needs to do to conform to management or funding expectations, often reducing complexity into statistics or milestones of dubious value. From this viewpoint, there is a resistance to evaluation because it appears to be more about control or compliance than enquiry or curiosity. Evaluation might also be seen to be over-academic, failing to capture the spirit and purpose of neighbourhood work.

Where neighbourhood work is sponsored directly or indirectly by major public bodies such as local authorities or health agencies, evaluation has often been reduced to nothing more than monitoring, associated with accountability and risk avoidance as much as with cost-effectiveness. Staff members are required to enter information about the people they have worked with, what they have done and how much time they have spent on each of the various activities specified in their work programme. Little is required or recorded, however, on the impact of these activities or how neighbourhoods may have benefited or changed. The local authority can access information if it is challenged and can provide a wealth of information about how much it has done. Whether such information provides valid evidence of community development is open to question.

There are also methodological and ethical difficulties in evaluation. The methodological ones revolve around the question of how you can measure processes or outcomes for concepts such as 'empowerment', 'engagement', 'resilience', 'capacity' or other intangibles that may be influenced by a whole range of factors beyond the control of the worker. The ethical issues centre on questions of intrusion and attribution:

- Evaluation can interfere with the activities of people and groups who have not necessarily agreed to be the focus of an evaluation: they simply want to achieve change in their community and do not see why 'they' should be evaluated.
- If a community group is successful, to what extent is that success attributable to its members' skills and hard work, as distinct from the competence of the worker or project that has supported them, or indeed to the attitude and responsiveness of other stakeholders? This is a difficult issue as direct attribution is impossible in a complex, fluid and changing environment. Nevertheless, a sensitive, questioning awareness to the factors that can be identified as having led to change (or resisted change) can provide useful clues about the impact that any activity may have had.

Such questions highlight the extent to which the outcomes of neighbourhood work may be difficult to compute and attribute. But this does not mean that useful information cannot be provided for evaluation. There are ways in which the three main concerns of neighbourhood work – community conditions, community engagement and community capacity – can be evaluated.

Community conditions can be assessed by the application of standardised and tested models. GoWell, the longitudinal study of well-being in different neighbourhoods in Glasgow, does this. Although community conditions rather than the processes of development are the focus, it gives a reliable and robust way of comparing conditions between neighbourhoods (www.gowellonline.com.uk). The New Economics Foundation offers a toolkit for social enterprises, using sets of indicators for social capital and community needs (www.neweconomics.org).

Community engagement can be understood as the nature and quality of relationships between

- community groups and neighbourhoods they are rooted in;
- neighbourhoods and public services.

Such engagement can be assessed and measured. In Scotland, the National Standards for Community Engagement, published by the Scottish Community Development Centre in 2005, sets out ten key areas for engagement practice and suggest indicators for assessing them all. These are indicators that can be used by both community and agency participants to hold each other to account on the core elements of engagement, including involving the right people, working collaboratively, planning inclusively and feeding back results and learning.

Each of these frameworks can be adapted to gauge the nature and function of any neighbourhood. In themselves, frameworks do not help to illuminate the choices the practitioner must make between balancing 'process' and 'task', between working with specific groups or across a whole neighbourhood. Nevertheless, an understanding of the nature and prospects for a neighbourhood is a good starting point for considering what areas to focus on and where to begin.

The choices to be made are founded on a recognition that neighbourhoods that have the ability can make things happen in a variety of ways. But there is often a choice to be made about which way may be best. Some things are better done within the neighbourhood through informal exchange between people with similar experiences or needs. This approach is sometimes described as self-help and is the basis of a great deal of community activity and interest.

Other situations are better addressed through some form of engagement between the neighbourhood and (usually) a relevant public service. In such circumstances there may be a shared concern about a community issue, a dialogue between the neighbourhood and the service about what might be done, and some form of collaboration in bringing it about. In the past this has been described as a social planning approach: these days it is more likely to be called engagement or co-production – by the public bodies if not by the community.

The third broad approach, closely aligned with some of the more radical models of neighbourhood work, is contest and campaigning. This is where community interests are threatened by some development or circumstance over which the community has no control. There appears to be no alternative other than to protest, lobby and mobilise for a change in the situation. Those who hold power will be unlikely to engage in a co-production approach in such circumstances, so the community is on its own and must build up its own alliances for change.

Although each of these approaches is of direct benefit to the community involved, it is also important to recognise that they may equally be of benefit to public services. Neighbourhoods that are well organised and inclusive are better equipped to engage in discussions about the way services can best be designed and delivered. They are also well placed to participate in decisions about development and change, and potentially be in a good position to contract for services that might otherwise be provided by the public sector. This should be taken into account when designing evaluation of neighbourhood work.

Useful tools and methods are available. The challenge is to make these meaningful and mainstream, and to assist the neighbourhood worker to make informed choices about which course of action to pursue.

Some principles

In an environment of monitoring and evaluation systems that do not accurately reflect the purpose of neighbourhood work (and might not give sufficient credit to its values), is there a more appropriate approach? We suggest that such an approach should be 'owned' by the field itself:

- The approach should be rooted in the values that underpin practice.
- It should focus on the core purposes and outcomes of the activity itself and not on its wider effects (although these do certainly need to be well understood and expressed).
- It should recognise and allow for complexity and the unexpected.

In Chapter 1, we refer to the values framework of the International Association for Community Development. To apply these values to evaluation means several things. First, the criteria for evaluation and the methods to be deployed should be negotiated in the neighbourhood, thereby avoiding imposing indicators or methods imported from elsewhere. The main purpose of evaluation is to ascertain the effect of action on matters that demand attention. Accordingly it should provide a basis for learning within the neighbourhood and thus be an important contributor to community empowerment, helping people acquire and improve their understanding, skills and confidence. This means it should pay close attention to qualitative factors as well as quantitative measures, ensuring some balance between the two.

Participative approaches designed along these principles can be empowering in themselves as they engage people directly in discussions and ownership of what the matters of concern are, what can be done about them, and who should be involved.

Second, evaluation appropriate to neighbourhood work should adopt a needs-led and outcome-focused approach. This invites a broad consideration of how things are and how they could be, rather than a narrow conception of what to do in the here-and-now situation with whatever resources happen to be available – described as the resource-led approach. As a simple example, a community-run centre adopting a resource-led approach might decide to organise drop-in tea and chat sessions for older residents to meet the centre's stated objective of encouraging more neighbourliness, reducing loneliness and increasing use of the facility.

An outcome-led approach, on the other hand, would seek to understand who in the neighbourhood was isolated, how they felt about it and what sort of response they would value and might get involved with personally. From this, a desired community outcome of greater interaction and exchange between different groups might be formulated. Then there might be an assessment of the obstacles to this being achieved. This could be followed by an understanding of the factors that may have led to the levels of loneliness experienced. From here, there could be a series of actions which, taken together, would be likely to increase connections between people. The tea and chat sessions could well be part of this but would not be the whole answer. If the actions were put in place they would be much more likely to engage their members in active roles such as making the tea, deciding on activities and getting involved in other things.

Thinking about outcomes in this way encourages a more engaging and participative exploration of people's experiences and ambitions. It involves people more directly in working for change and recognises that many factors may need attention if lasting change is to occur.

Evaluation in practice

We now turn to considering how a neighbourhood worker might best approach the task of evaluation. We want to distinguish this from how a funder or policy manager might undertake the same task. For the funder or policy manager, evaluation questions are typically framed around whether a practitioner has met certain set targets or has achieved value for money. These questions are also important for the neighbourhood worker but are less important than the question of the impact the work is having, and the lessons to be learned to further develop the worker's skills.

For the neighbourhood worker, the first priority is to pose and address significant questions about her work and its relevance to the neighbourhood. This means that she should become comfortable with the idea of critical reflection and performance assessment that is focused on her own practice, in other words embedding evaluation in all aspects of her work as a matter of course. This may appear burdensome and may be subject to criticisms of bias or subjectivity. But if it is seen as a necessary part of good practice in an uncertain and changing environment, it can be an excellent way of imposing coherence and direction over how the environment might be best understood as the context of practice. Although self-evaluation is primarily for the benefit of the practitioner, it remains the case that a robust approach to self-evaluation will also provide strong and substantiated evidence of impact whenever an external evaluation is called for.

We would like to convey the idea that self-evaluation should become normal – part of the stock in trade of the reflective practitioner who should always have a curious and critical approach to what she does and be motivated to hone and own her practice.

Such a practitioner will always have a set of searching questions near the front of her mind, especially the extent to which she is gaining a sound understanding of community needs and issues. Is she being effective in tackling them, and is she being inclusive and encouraging others to be so? Another key issue to consider concerns the neighbourhood: is it achieving its goals and is the worker helping it to build and make use of its assets and resources? The practitioner should address the question of community learning: is the work empowering people and building neighbourhood skills and knowledge? Not only will she be learning but the community should be, too. A culture of collaboration, participation and sustainable change should underpin neighbourhood work. And at the heart of this is the challenge of whether actions taken are contributing to the well-being and quality of life of most residents. Finally, addressing the issues of resources and evidence are critical: is best use of the resources to hand being made, and is the evidence available which is needed to inform and influence future decisions? These questions are at the heart of reflective community development practice.

A good working knowledge of the contents of this book will assist greatly in addressing these questions. In addition, a cognitive map or mental picture of neighbourhood work and the processes involved will be of value. The skills and methods described here can be understood as ways in which the worker can help bring about two distinct but related sets of outcomes. These can be seen as the 'community empowerment' and 'quality of community life' components of neighbourhood work. These two concepts underpin the publication by Barr and Hashagen (2000) on which the remainder of this chapter draws directly.

Community empowerment

There are four spheres which can be understood as the essential 'community empowerment' outcomes from effective neighbourhood work. These are personal empowerment, positive action, community organisation, and participation and involvement. We describe each in the following:

Personal empowerment: neighbourhood work is fundamentally about developing skills, confidence, understanding and self-esteem through people getting involved, taking action, participating with others and reflection. Such learning applies individually and collectively so that both individuals and groups have a greater ability to achieve change. A core purpose of neighbourhood work is to encourage such learning, recognising that there can be many obstacles to personal empowerment. Some people experience such disadvantage and discrimination that they live their lives in a dependent or alienated way and do not perceive the possibility of change. Others may believe there is no point in trying to change things, or would leave it to others, believing that they lack the skills or confidence to take action themselves. Or they may fear that by taking action they would be laying themselves open to sanctions or punishment by more powerful forces.

These forces all conspire against disadvantaged or excluded communities promoting their own interests. It is for this reason that community development, and much of its theory, starts with the question of how to empower people to take action.

Positive action: inequalities in resource allocation and power are a key reason for investment in neighbourhood work. Known inequalities between groups, a lack of cohesion and disaffection are concerns both within communities and in public discourse. Neighbourhood work has an important role to play in community building and increasing social capital as discussed in the previous chapter. We can use the term positive action to convey the sum of meanings included in the concepts of equal opportunity, social justice, social inclusion and anti-discriminatory practice. The idea of positive action is fundamental to community development because the source of obstacles to community change and progress lies in obstacles/barriers and imbalances in access to power, to being heard, or in active discrimination against certain groups. Change should build on an acceptance and understanding of others. Exclusion on the grounds of disability, race, gender or sexual orientation has already been discussed. It is also important to recognise that people may also be excluded by poverty, culture or the actions of public policy. Exclusion may also operate within communities. Some community leaders may represent their constituencies without any form of accountability to them or may try to maintain one set of values against another ('I speak for the respectable members of this community . . .'). The key to understanding positive action is to recognise the barriers and biases inherent in systems of power, dominance and subservience, and to seek to challenge, overcome or dismantle them.

Community organisation: neighbourhood work is also about organising – creating structures and infrastructures that can give support and solidarity, lobby for change, provide meaningful and valued services or which can work with others. Again, outcomes can be set, worked towards and measured.

A central purpose of neighbourhood work is to strengthen the range and quality of social life and collective activity in communities. This works at several levels, from simple exchanges such as keeping an eye on neighbours' homes while they are away, or perhaps helping older people with shopping or gardening, or lending tools or DVDs. Such activities may become a little more organised – involving, for example, shopping for people who are extremely vulnerable to COVID-19, babysitting circles, mother and toddler groups or neighbourhood watch schemes – to a higher level. Then there are groups that exist to identify and represent community needs and issues, which may include school boards, neighbourhood forums or tenants' associations. More formal community-led organisations may emerge. They may employ staff, have buildings or other assets, and offer a range of services or activities in communities. Examples include community-run housing associations, development trusts and independent living centres. At a broader level still, there are organisations within the community sector that serve to represent common interests or provide services to members or networks. All these levels of organisation can be nurtured and supported through neighbourhood work activity.

Participation and involvement: all these spheres contribute to the efficacy of a neighbourhood – in other words its ability to influence decisions, represent community opinion and interests, and generally shape the development of the neighbourhood.

Neighbourhood work has a role to play in encouraging and supporting this. The sphere of participation and influence is where the empowered community interacts with the outside world to achieve change. In planning community development, and in evaluating it, it is thus crucial to:

- understand the relationships between communities and those political and administrative systems providing services;
- look at how neighbourhoods go about working for change;
- consider the obstacles and opportunities that exist.

Agencies that are committed to using a community development approach must also consider how they go about maximising the opportunities for neighbourhoods to participate and have influence over the way they work.

The four spheres described earlier can be seen as the essential building blocks of community empowerment. They are the basis on which neighbourhoods can get to the point where they can participate actively in their own development. They are the preconditions for engagement. Given that the core purpose of neighbourhood work is to strengthen and sustain these pillars, it is important to have ways to assess progress and change.

Quality of community life

The quality of community life outcomes is the change in community conditions and well-being, which can generally be understood as the 'tasks' that is required to bring about community change. In Chapter 5 we explore the kinds of needs that may be of concern in a neighbourhood, around which community groups focus their attention and energy. Such needs and issues can be broadly grouped into five themes or 'outcome areas':

Working community: There has been a long tradition of community economic development in many countries. In the United Kingdom, the United States and Ireland, community businesses were established from the mid-1970s, while since the 1980s much of the force of regeneration has been directed to creating jobs and training for those excluded from the labour market. This thinking has persisted, and in more recent years has linked up with the other arm of community economic activity – anti-poverty and welfare rights campaigns. There are now community organisations which are an important part of their local economies, providing services, offering alternatives or encouraging access. Examples include development trusts, community businesses, credit unions, Local Exchange Trading Schemes (LETs), debt counselling and money advice and community-based housing associations.

Such community-led organisations all seek to increase incomes, to reduce costs or to expand the number and range of assets within community control. Other initiatives, such as community transport schemes or food co-operatives, may have environmental or social benefit, and also serve to reduce costs. All such initiatives have the potential to become community enterprises. Thus community economic development can combat poverty and exclusion and reduce inequality and division.

Caring community: One of the most important characteristics of a strong community is the kind of support and care it offers its members. Older people, disabled people, lone parents and carers often depend on the support that is available within a neighbourhood. There may be many levels of activity in communities that support people informally and complement the services available from the state. The latter's services may be increasingly difficult to access in times of economic hardship. It is also the case that much of the focus of participation and influence is on the nature and quality of social service provision. In this dimension of the quality of life, however, we are essentially looking at the nature and extent of those services that support and sustain people's lives in communities.

Safe community: The stimulus for much community action has been a real or perceived threat to the health or safety of people living in neighbourhoods. It is important to be aware that poor neighbourhoods are not just where poor people happen to live. They are almost invariably the least safe, least healthy, least stimulating environments, and the motivation to deal with these fears and dangers is the motivation behind everything from neighbourhood watch schemes, through protests against industrial pollution to running voluntary after-school care schemes.

Creative community: The bonds that build communities are as much about shared experience, celebration and culture as about economics, environment or services. It is part of all traditional cultures and communities that there are shared celebrations to mark the change in seasons, historical events or the religious calendar. Arts and drama are used and can become a valuable method of helping communities identify and express issues and needs. The nature, variety and significance given to this are therefore an important part of community development and of the quality of neighbourhood life. We take a broad view of the notion of a 'creative community' and include within it all forms of festivals, arts, sports and spiritual activity.

Citizen's community: There is no real point to neighbourhood work unless change is involved. The emphasis on how communities can develop the capacity to influence change effectively is fundamental. However, as well as being a process of empowerment, the context of political expression is an important component of the quality of community life. Although we may all live in a democracy with policy-making being a product of a recognised political process, the way that is experienced will vary widely. Some government activities will go much further than others in engaging the public in debating and developing policy, and the same is true of local government, non-elected boards and, indeed, voluntary organisations. Community development emphasises the values of openness, dialogue, inclusion and participation, and the quality of community life is enhanced where these values are embedded in local cultures and relationships.

Overall, neighbourhood work is founded on the assumption that people want to live in healthy, well-functioning neighbourhoods. These are communities in which people feel able to be who they are, have good prospects and experience respect, as well as equal and fair treatment in all spheres of life. The purpose of neighbourhood work is primarily to focus on places where such characteristics are lacking, and to help bring about change.

We can take the themes described earlier both as the essential areas of concern for neighbourhood work and as outcome areas – in other words the domains in which change may be expected and measured. Understood in this way, they describe in broad terms the benefits that should be expected and evident from the activity and which should therefore be subject to evaluation. To go back to our key questions concerning measurement, intrusion and attribution, a critical appraisal of progress in each outcome area should provide useful information from which the questions can be answered.

The language of evaluation

The neighbourhood worker needs a basic understanding of the language and concept of evaluation. Particularly important are the ideas of inputs, processes, outputs and outcomes. Each of these is central to good planning, and consequently equally important to evaluation.

- *Inputs* in relation to neighbourhood work are the resources available, and may include funds, equipment, spaces, information, time, energy and many other tangible or intangible assets.
- *Processes* are in essence actions: things that are done using the available resources with the intention of leading towards some desired outcome. They include organising, mediating, representing, motivating, meditating and other types of action considered in later chapters. They are the skills that the worker needs to have and to enhance through actions and learning.
- *Outputs* are the direct product of the processes, and may be a survey report, a new group or service, a community arts festival, a plan or an organised protest against a proposed development. They are within the direct control of those responsible for their preparation and provision.
- *Outcomes* are the desired future state of affairs that the outputs are designed to bring about. The outcomes from the outputs described earlier might respectively be greater awareness about community circumstances and motivation to act; more fun, learning and interaction between young and old; a sense of clarity, purpose and feasibility; and the reversal of a development decision. Outcomes, however, are not within the control of whoever provided the output: they can be and will be subject to many other factors some of which will be well outside the influence of those directly involved.

Each of these components can be evaluated to gain an understanding of their significance to any activity. The inputs may be sufficient and available to support the action, or they may not. Processes – the methods and skills of the worker and the other players – can be examined for their contribution. Outputs may succeed, or they may not. A public meeting, which attracts only a handful of people, and where the key speaker is boring or irrelevant, can be evaluated, as can one with an enthusiastic attendance and an energising speaker. It should go without saying that the quality of the output is mainly in the hands of the organiser – a failure often means there has been insufficient attention to the need, purpose and expected outcome. This brings us back to the importance of the expected outcome from any activity.

As we described earlier, neighbourhood work is best conducted when a consideration of outcomes is the first step – what is it that needs to improve or change? Wherever possible, outcomes should be based on a clear understanding of needs and issues, and their definition will derive from a vision shared with, or generated by, local people. To construct a useful evaluation model, we need to have measures or indicators – evidence that can tell us something about what is happening, what is changing, and why. Bringing all this together, we can establish a model that will help plan, evaluate and learn from any neighbourhood work initiative. The model is most helpfully thought of as a series of questions, and looks like this:

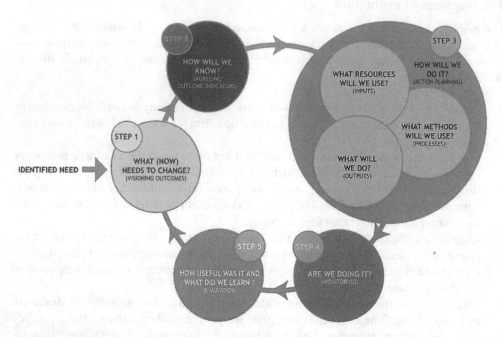

Figure 2.1 The LEAP planning and evaluation cycle
Source: NHS Scotland, 2003: 19

Figure 2.1 is not only about evaluation, but also about the basis of planning decisions and evaluation questions. As such it requires the ability to understand the nature of the neighbourhood, how people feel about it and how motivated they may be to get involved. We will need to know what the local issues and concerns are, who has identified them and whether these perceptions are widely shared. We may also need to examine why we should get involved in the neighbourhood in the first place.

The reader will find a great deal of detail in the book about how to understand the nature of a neighbourhood, clarifying problems and issues, prioritising between options and working with people towards better outcomes. For the purposes of evaluation, we need some accessible and dependable information that will allow us to make judgements on the extent to which the outcomes have been achieved. The factors that can be looked at to enable us to make such judgements are called indicators, or measures. Some of these can be quantifiable, such as the number of people attending a public meeting, the numbers in receipt of additional benefits as a result of a claims campaign, or young people moving into employment from a community-based skills training course. Such information is clearly useful but can mask the actual value of the activity to those involved. So we really need to know the extent to which the people who attended the meeting got anything out of it, whether the increased income made the community as a whole more financially self-reliant, or whether the skills gained by the young people benefited the community in some way. So as well as quantifiable indicators, we need qualitative ones that will help understand whether the neighbourhood is becoming better organised, more equal, more cohesive or more assertive.

The following are some examples of indicators which relate to the primary goals of neighbourhood work. In a 'developed' neighbourhood:

- community groups act as leaders and drivers for local change through their own activities and through their influence on others;
- they are recognised by the local community as legitimate and accountable representatives;
- there is a community culture of confidence, assertiveness and competence;
- community groups actively reach out to engage and involve all members of the community, in particular those usually viewed or perceived as excluded;
- community groups and public agencies jointly reflect on and learn from planned activity and its impact on change in the community.

Conversely, in a neighbourhood where intervention is needed:

- there are few community groups and those that exist are isolated or in competition with others, operate unilaterally or lack leadership;
- the neighbourhood suffers from the actions of outside interests and is unable to defend its position or influence what happens;
- groups are resistant to the idea of learning or skill development;
- there is a breakdown of trust between different interest groups; excluded groups are denied a voice and are actively excluded from community activity and decisions;
- community groups have disengaged from decision-making completely, due to negative experiences.

Clearly there can be no specific quantifiable measures of such factors, but in going through the processes described in the chapters that follow, the worker will be able to get a sense of where things stand on these and other factors. This can be checked out and refined through the conversations he or she has, and can be recorded as the 'baseline' situation. The same questions can be asked again at later intervals and any improvements in the situation recorded. Such improvement can then be attributed, at least in part, to the neighbourhood work activities that have taken place. Returning to the principles of collaboration and participation as the core values of neighbourhood work, the more that local people can be involved in specifying outcomes, defining indicators that are relevant to them and taking part in gathering information and evidence the better. It is more likely that the evaluation will reflect the real ambitions and perspectives of the neighbourhood.

The indicators described earlier relate to the capacity building role that is central to neighbourhood work. Indicator sets for many other elements of community development are available, for instance:

- Leap for Health for community health improvement;
- in relation to Scotland, the National Standards for Community Engagement, and VOiCE which covers the same territory in an online format;
- the Social Capital Toolkit, for social capital and health;
- Greenspace LEAP framework for community environmental action;
- LEAP core texts and LEAP online.

All of these can be accessed via the SCDC website (www.scdc.org.uk).

Plans and processes

Once we have our outcomes and indicators in place, we can consider how we might best go about achieving the outcomes. This is essentially the planning process, and it involves three main considerations: the resources to hand, the methods available and the actions to be put in place. How can we deploy each of these to best effect in bringing about the outcomes we seek? There is much advice on these questions throughout the book, and workers have to apply their own experience in deciding how to proceed in any given situation. The key questions do, however, remain the same:

- Which course of action is most likely to lead to the desired outcomes, bearing in mind the principles of social justice, involvement and empowerment?
- Is it necessary to do this, and will it be sufficient?
- Will this be *effective*, will it be *efficient* and will it respect *equalities*?

In other words will it work, will it be cost-effective and will it benefit those in greatest need?

The planning process should culminate in an action plan: what is going to happen or be done; when it is going to happen; who is to be responsible and how it is going to work. The 'why' question should already have been asked and answered: it will have been decided as the most effective, efficient and equality-aware way of reaching the desired outcome. With such an action plan in place, it can be relatively easy to keep track of how things are progressing – this is usually known as *monitoring*. For every output, monitoring seeks to establish whether:

- it took place as it was intended to;
- it was successful in its own terms;
- any future action needs to be adjusted in light of this scrutiny.

The evaluation forms often circulated at events are a good way of getting useful feedback (if the questions are posed carefully), and a debrief session involving everyone with an interest in the activity can also prove invaluable.

When all these components are in place, the worker, community groups, funder or programme manager will be in a good position to conduct an evaluation. They will have the information and evidence they need, and there will be a good, shared understanding of the outcomes desired, the quality of the inputs, the relevance of the processes and the way the outputs were received. In many neighbourhoods, a well-conducted self-evaluation can provide invaluable evidence for an external evaluation and can be a significant part of the process. With all the evidence to hand, and ideally with all the people with an interest in the matter gathered together, the key questions for evaluation can be addressed. In doing so, other important questions which may well be posed are as follows:

- Do you have the information you need?
- What have you learned about the methods chosen and ability to work with them?
- Have actions been well planned, has good advice, support and guidance been offered, how have obstacles been dealt with?
- What have you learned about the inputs?

- What about the theory? Did actions lead to outcomes? What were the success factors? What was learned?
- What has been the impact? What has been the evidence of change in cultures, the environment and quality of life? How much can be attributed to the work – what would/would not have happened without it? Have there been any unintended consequences?
- Has the project been efficient, effective and equitable?

Once these questions have been addressed and explored, all concerned will have a good understanding about what went right and what went wrong:

- Did the desired change happen?
- Have other unanticipated changes taken place?
- Have people become involved in unexpected ways or gone on to new challenges?

Many useful insights and issues may emerge and these can become a fundamental part of how the neighbourhood sees itself and understands the progress it is making. Such reflection is invaluable and should rightly be celebrated. Lessons will have been learned, the dynamics of the neighbourhood better understood, and the potential and limitations of change more fully recognised. All this learning can then be usefully applied to the important question of 'what next?' On the basis of the new understanding of issues, needs and opportunities, the question of 'what needs to change' can be reconsidered: it becomes 'what now needs to change?' and involves a refreshed consideration of possibilities, vision and ambition.

These guidelines on evaluation should enable neighbourhood workers, in partnership with their managers and local people, to ensure that planning and evaluation are integral to neighbourhood work practice. In the appendix we provide an example of a project using the LEAP framework. In the next chapter we begin our presentation of the neighbourhood work process by examining the opening moves of the neighbourhood worker.

References

Barr, A. and Hashagen, S. (2000) *ABCD handbook. A framework for evaluating community development*, London: CDF Publications.

Christie, C. (2011) *Commission on the future delivery of public services*, Edinburgh: The Scottish Government. Online. Available HTTP: <www.scotland.gov.uk/Publications.2011.06/27154527/0)> (accessed 23 April 2012).

Health Empowerment Leverage Project. (2011) *Empowering communities for health: business case and practice framework*. Online. Available HTTP: <www.healthempowermentgroup.org.uk> (accessed 19 February 2012).

3   Entering the neighbourhood

Thinking about going in	Negotiating entry
Orientation	Existing community groups
Values and roles	Agencies
Planning and problem analysis	The worker's agency

How a worker starts the succession of steps, which gains him or her access to a neighbourhood, is of critical importance. The 'way in' has to be thought through rigorously because of the commitments and pressures that will inevitably build up. It is also when neighbourhood workers may need to have intensive support from colleagues and supervisors.

This chapter examines the kind of preliminary thinking and action which needs to take place. We call these *thinking about going in* and *negotiating entry*. All of it is still very much in the pre-action phase of neighbourhood work. The question of whether a practitioner will 'go in' at all to a neighbourhood remains legitimate and relevant throughout.

Thinking about going in

The motivation to throw yourself quickly into some form of practical activity is normally strong. This is true both of practitioners newly appointed to posts and of established practitioners starting projects in a neighbourhood where they have not worked before. The expression and satisfaction of the 'doing' of neighbourhood work, compared with thinking and talking about it, entice even the most experienced practitioners to move rapidly into seeking out and working with people.

In many respects this tendency is as unsurprising as it is welcome: workers who are not eager about finding out how people express community needs, or who do not genuinely enjoy working closely with a multiplicity and variety of local people, are unlikely to stay with neighbourhood work for long. The themes of felt and expressed needs and of working alongside people, rather than simply on their behalf, lie at the heart of a worker's involvement in the neighbourhood.

The stage before contact begins consists of a combination of orientation by the worker to his or her surroundings and of building up a plan of entry into the neighbourhood. It involves avoiding making decisions too early on while at the same time maintaining antennae which are constantly alert to useful information, leads, contacts and potential allies.

DOI: 10.4324/9781003310006-3

The questions which the worker needs to have at the front of his or her mind at this stage are: What kind of work should I do? What are the best ways of helping me do it? How should I set about getting there? The formulation of such questions is an essential antecedent for practitioners and the teams of which they are members. An important influence on the formulation of questions should be a practitioner's thinking about what he or she learnt from the last job, project or campaign, although this should be done critically – practitioners can get 'stuck' with an early success and keep trying to repeat it. We distinguish the following as being central to a practitioner's consideration: *orientation, values and roles* and *planning and problem analysis*.

Orientation

Neighbourhood workers inevitably have to know and work with a range of professionals, in varied organisational settings. The nature of their work forces them into this position. They will usually need to know, and be known by, many organisations and individuals in the areas where they work. They tend to become walking encyclopaedias of relevant, up-to-date information about who's who and where to go in the neighbourhoods and in the organisations that serve them.

Anyone who intends to become seriously involved in a neighbourhood must set time aside for absorbing the nature of the neighbourhood and the attitudes and interests of both local people and professional colleagues. The practitioner can always correct and improve initial impressions later. The importance of this initial scanning lies in awakening the worker's senses to the number and range of factors to be considered before moving into action. Orientation thus becomes an essential preliminary to planning intervention in the neighbourhood.

As far as the community aspect is concerned, it can mean simply walking about an area – a stranger literally taking the first steps towards eventual partnership with local people. It is best if workers vary the times of the day and night at which they make such forays, for then they will be more likely to absorb an accurate, albeit sketchy, picture. When workers engage in such walking about, they must be careful not to confuse it with more detailed and deliberate observation and contact-making in the community, both of which are distinct phases which come later. The worker's incursions into the community at this stage are to assist in deciding how to plan an intervention; they come strictly in the pre-planning phase.

Characteristics of the neighbourhood to be noticed are degrees of traffic densities in different streets; condition and types of housing; the extent of untidiness and vandalism; the existence of open space; the location of factories, offices and pubs; places of worship and shops, and the availability of public transport. The worker might note, too, some obvious features about people in the area: older people walking uphill with their shopping, the presence of young people, or simply the ebb and flow of people at different times of the day.

Some of the impressions will merely reaffirm what the worker has been told already by colleagues, while others will be new; it will depend a lot on whether the worker is starting a new piece of work in the area, or whether he or she is joining an existing programme for which there are background papers and reports. Whether the messages a worker receives are old or new when she familiarises herself with the area and with the lifestyles of its residents, they form a key part of the worker's orientation.

The effort of tuning into the organisational context of the job demands, first of all, that practitioners begin to obtain a grasp of agency functioning. They will usually start with their own agency and then broaden out to acquire an initial understanding of organisations which either operate alongside their own agency or which they know are likely to impinge in some way on the neighbourhood where they intend to work. There are a number of further actions that practitioners need to take in relation to organisations, which we discuss later in the chapter.

A final component of the orientation phase incorporates both the community and the agency: an awareness of the social, economic and political climate in which the practitioner is to practise neighbourhood work. Two contrasting examples:

• The regional community development organisation in Brussels, SAAMO, takes the lead in innovative housing projects such as 'Solidar Mobiel Wonen' in the neighbourhood of Magritte. Homeless men were involved with the project from the beginning. Architectural students and the homeless men visited and scanned a number of areas. They listened to residents' comments and suggestions and decided on Magritte. Plans were drawn up for eight housing units. The SAAMO community workers organised a dialogue with the local council and the Brussels authority. Both of these agreed to the setting up of a pilot project and the community workers began to involve the residents: 'The interaction with the neighbourhood is crucial for the integration of the newcomers in this housing project' (Hautekeur, personal communication).

• In Northern Ireland an experienced community worker returned to the community on Lough Neagh, where he was brought up, and began a small woodworking business. He encouraged people to use the workshop and he set up woodwork classes. From this experience there developed an interest in local history and, with the encouragement of the Workers Educational Association, speakers were invited – an old shed was renovated as a venue – and at the same time people were encouraged to tell their own stories. We have described how this community worker began his involvement because it points to the advantages of beginning slowly and carefully to encourage communication and participation among rural people (Francis and Henderson, 1992: 110–111).

It is possible for a worker to identify sets of attitudes that permeate the area where he or she is due to work. The urban/rural contrast will be one determinant, as will the overall extent of relative affluence or deprivation. As each day passes, the worker will be adding to his or her store of knowledge on these and other points, tightening up initial perceptions or assumptions. At some point the worker is likely to want to set time aside for methodical study of some of these by, for example, examination of an area's social history. In the initial stages, however, the worker should be ready to receive the hidden messages and assumptions in the community and its institutions, exploring political, social and economic complexities. This is likely to help workers to pitch the character and form of their interventions in a neighbourhood at the right level. It will be particularly relevant for when they first approach existing community groups. What the worker sees, and the interpretations he or she makes, will inevitably be subjective at this stage. Equally, first impressions will not always be entirely accurate. It will also be important for a worker to be aware of impressions that residents may have of an incoming worker, particularly if she is new to the area.

Values and roles

When planning interventions in a neighbourhood, workers need to spend time clarifying their own position on key value issues. The decisions they take once they move into a neighbourhood will be partly determined by their values and by their perception of role. They must have a stance on both of these and be ready to articulate them when necessary. Several of the contributors to *Building Practitioner Strengths* draw attention to this imperative, for example:

> Gee's motivation and commitment to community development is based upon her strong value base and sense of injustice and inequality. Her starting point is local people and the need to 'get out there' and above all 'listen'. It's about making contacts, building up relationships and finding out what the issues of concern are to local people.
>
> (Wilson and Wilde, 2001: 52)

We shall do no more here than list five issues that relate to values and role. Our prime interest is to identify some of the relevant questions to be aware of before the worker starts to make contact with the community. There are several others, and they are bound to vary in significance for each person.

Process/product

A continuing dilemma is whether your interest lies essentially in assisting the self-learning process of individuals through their participation in community groups, or whether it focuses more on the achievement of specific tasks which can bring material or psychological benefits to neighbourhoods. This does not have to be a dichotomy. If workers favour a combination of the two, how do they attempt to maintain a balance, and how do they handle the difficulties which arise when process and product goals come into conflict – as they will do sometimes? The worker has to see the intricate connection between the two. Closely linked to this question is that of timescale, of how long or short a time commitment a worker will make to a neighbourhood. Often this is not within his or her control, because of being part of a team which will be subject to management decisions; also, because the worker's activities will be target or outcome driven. However, whatever the context may be, the balancing and integrating of the connections and tensions between process and product need to be addressed.

Consideration of these questions implies, in effect, that a practitioner should have conceptualised a philosophy and set of objectives for working at neighbourhood level. It should include analysis of the links that neighbourhood work can make between local, national and global issues, between his or her involvement in practice at neighbourhood level and the wider social, economic and environmental policies that affect the locality.

Skills and craft

It is tempting to suggest that some practitioners, when planning to enter a neighbourhood, have a natural instinct to follow the right paths. They appear to handle neighbourhood work as a craft rather than as a skill that has been learned. While we think it is unhelpful to make too strong a distinction between the two concepts, there do seem to be practitioners who can act intuitively. There are few of them and even the most naturally gifted would be unlikely to decry the usefulness of training, guidance and planning. Most neighbourhood practitioners need to acquire a number of skills and develop particular qualities in order to be effective in their work. Furthermore, they depend on being able to use analytic tools and a rational process to assist them in their tasks. Before they start working in a neighbourhood, it is probably helpful for practitioners to assess where they put themselves on a continuum stretching from acquired skills to simply having the knack or intuition.

The style in which they operate will affect the kind of projects workers choose to develop, as well as the support mechanisms they will require. They need to have an idea of their own strengths and weaknesses as individuals if they are to perform effectively; all workers make abundant use of themselves as people and of the human qualities they possess. Furthermore, workers may have to develop aspects of their personality for the benefit of their work which they may never have used before.

Participation

It is recognised that theories of participation are of direct relevance to neighbourhood workers, with the proviso that involving large numbers of people is not always appropriate or sufficient for bringing about major changes in a community. A worker may often be forced to choose between the effectiveness of a small group of people working on a task, set against an awareness of the importance of expanding such a group's membership. The worker has to be aware of this potential disjunction of aims, which he or she is likely to face frequently. One criterion that can be used is the degree to which a group's membership is added to and renewed. Groups with small membership may still represent a constituency, but groups that consist of self-perpetuating cliques have moved a long way from the participatory goals of community work.

Leadership

Neighbourhood workers are rapidly put in the position of having to accept, deflect or reject requests to them from individuals and groups in the community to take on leadership roles. While neighbourhood work aims to enable local people to assume leadership in a multiplicity of situations, it may be appropriate to the methods and strategies of a neighbourhood worker for him or her to play a leadership role as an interim measure. We shall suggest that this is particularly likely in situations where the formation of a group is difficult and time-consuming, and where a worker can legitimately demonstrate leadership skills or give confidence to a group by providing it with direction.

Since workers can safely anticipate being put under pressure to provide leadership, it is necessary for them to crystallise their response beforehand. The same applies to the style of work they intend to adopt and the role they favour (we examine these in detail in Chapter 5). When they change role, it is important to convey a clear impression of who they are, what they are bringing to the work and what they will be doing. This area is particularly important when the diversity of the membership of many community groups is considered.

Accountability

In the event of a conflict of interest arising between a worker's agency and a group he or she supports, the worker needs to have ready a set of arguments to underpin whatever position is taken. Even when no conflict arises, a worker will usually experience tension between his or her agency and the community's interests, although this will vary according to the kind of agency in which someone is employed. For example, a worker is always aware of the danger of giving away too much information to power-holders about community groups and how they work.

The question of accountability of workers relates closely to the ethics of intervention in a community. Both are issues which workers have to think about carefully. It is certain that the rigour and clarity of the thinking will be put to the test in the work situation; it is exceptional for neighbourhood workers to remain onlookers.

It is worth noting again that most workers will find themselves as members of an agency, a project or a community work team. Thus the worker will not have a blank cheque but will be held to account by other team members and managers.

In itemising the aforementioned issues surrounding the subjects of values and role, we emphasise again that we have sought only to identify key ideas and not to develop them. Their study and debate must form an essential part of any work in a neighbourhood, and our decision merely to list them should not be taken as undervaluing either their significance or their complexity.

Planning and problem analysis

It will be seen that the emphasis we give to planning entry into a neighbourhood is upon the value of reflection and orientation, especially in relation to a worker's values and role. It has to do with the nature of the work which is going to be undertaken, and the attitudes the worker takes with him or her when starting to know a neighbourhood. It is the stage in the neighbourhood work process when workers will have most time to think at this level without interruption and without being over-influenced by their involvement. Once they are working on projects and issues in the neighbourhood, the pressures of time and competing needs, demands and events will prejudice their ability to do such reflective thinking.

The development of a plan of entry must include what Ross (1967) calls 'the process of locating and defining a problem (or set of problems)'. It is important to stress the spiral-like movement of problem analysis and action, each being informed by the other as the work proceeds. The bursts of activity in neighbourhood work and the rapid accumulation of tasks, meetings and contacts can conceal attempts made deliberately to follow steps in a process, even if the steps cannot be sequential.

We agree, however, with Perlman and Gurin (1972) that 'organising people to achieve social change requires planning to guide both the ends and means of their efforts'. A major component in the worker's pre-planning phase is the identification of the categories of activities and tasks which have to be undertaken and which will enable the worker to begin building up a description of a neighbourhood's needs, assets and aspirations. The worker will then be in a position to analyse the problems, and from there formulate a plan of action.

Too close an equation of developing a plan of intervention with problem analysis of a neighbourhood carries with it a danger of implying entirely negative characteristics of the local environment and of the people who live there. Any such tendency should certainly be avoided. Neighbourhood workers try, above all, to seek out and nourish the strengths and resources of local communities and shun any suggestions of labelling.

Our argument up to this point is that neighbourhood workers, having spent time on reflection and orientation, have to begin to sharpen their ideas about what they intend to do. This can be achieved by them finding out and broadly categorising the problems facing a neighbourhood, and thence devising a plan of intervention. Closely linked to this is the need for workers to obtain initial legitimacy for their plans and future presence.

Negotiating entry

Neighbourhood workers sometimes use the device of involving themselves with short-term or relatively minor activities in a neighbourhood, such as a street party or a tidying up project, with the purpose of using them to open up contacts for working on more major issues and problems – it does not, of course, always work. This approach might be called the direct way into working with the community. While it can have distinct tactical advantages, we consider that, if it is not preceded or accompanied by more searching and explicit moves by the worker to begin the neighbourhood work process, it is likely to be counter-productive.

We call this work negotiating entry, and suggest that it can be differentiated from later steps of gathering data and building up contacts. Clearly, in negotiating entry, the worker does collect data and meet people. The chief difference is that, while the last two are related directly to engagement in a neighbourhood, negotiating entry is concerned with clearing a pathway which will facilitate that engagement.

Such an approach will be successful in many instances as a means of generating a work programme, and we shall see later (Chapter 6) how informal contact-making constitutes a crucial part of the worker's task once he or she has formulated a plan of action. We believe, however, that there are dangers in relying on it at an early stage in neighbourhood work. It reduces the possibility of the worker forming a reasonably accurate picture of the area, and the people and organisations in it, *before committing himself or herself to any action*. It can also distract workers from opening up communications with key agencies – including their own – which already have a presence in the area.

Furthermore, it is the experience of many practitioners that, once committed to a line of action with existing groups, or even with those in the process of formation, it becomes very difficult for them to draw back and start afresh with different groups or a new constituency. Too early an engagement may result in practitioners finding themselves supporting groups with which, at a later stage, they would prefer not to be so closely involved, or from which they would actually like to dissociate themselves.

In practice, the practitioner will frequently become involved with an existing community activity as a means of entering the community at the same time as drawing up an ordered and selected snapshot of the area as a prelude to formulating a plan. Or the practitioner will latch on to an obvious need which can begin to be met swiftly.

Kospallag is a settlement in Hungary of 800 inhabitants. Neighbourhood work started there by selecting an old farmhouse. This was done between a group of ethnographers invited by a community association, and the link quickly became one of friendship and collaboration. The project developed rapidly so that, in addition to renovating the house with traditional techniques, it came to include exploring the village's past and traditions. Learning about the relationship between the past and the present steered the team towards neighbourhood work, including identifying resources and responding to gaps (Vercseg, personal communication).

Negotiating entry demands rigorous thinking on the part of the worker along with some preliminary and minimal contact with community leaders and professional workers. We are conscious of the risk of being over-prescriptive in a field of activity which is characterised by great diversity. There may also be differences for a worker depending on whether she or he is employed by a statutory or voluntary organisation: someone employed in a small voluntary project may have more flexibility than a worker located in a large statutory organisation, and this kind of difference will shape the thinking and planning undertaken at this stage.

The role involves the following components:

- requesting and selecting information;
- giving information about the employing organisation;
- self-introduction and introduction of others;
- hearing and checking casual information such as gossip and rumour.

We shall now examine the extent to which workers use these and other skills, and how they do so in the three major arenas where they will do their work in this phase: existing community groups, relevant agencies and their own organisation.

Existing community groups

A worker may plan to operate in a neighbourhood where someone has not worked before, or may be due to enter an area which has already experienced the intervention of one or more neighbourhood workers or other community-based practitioners. Whichever it is, an awareness that boundaries are about to be crossed is essential. This is true in the psychological, political and geographical sense of boundary. Until a worker begins to gain the trust of individuals, families, existing leadership and groups in a community, he or she is as much an intruder there as any stranger would be. Writing about the difficulty of organising community groups, Jacobs comments that 'The poor have good reason to view representatives of the welfare state with deep suspicion, even when appearing in the apparently friendly guise of community worker' (Jacobs and Popple, 1994: 169).

When neighbourhood workers are planning a fresh piece of intervention, it is essential for them to be aware of existing social identities in neighbourhoods – how local people believe their community is perceived by others and the complex, diverse and dynamic nature of social identities. Attention is drawn to this point in order to underline the sensitivity and listening skills upon which neighbourhood workers have to draw as they start to discover the complex workings of a community and begin to obtain recognition from parts of it. Workers will be as much under observation, and being tested out, as observing and exploring the community themselves. Understanding how they are likely to be perceived and thinking carefully about how they present themselves will make a big difference to how easily they are able to build trust and develop relationships across the whole community. In particular, showing awareness of their own identity and respect for other cultures might mean acknowledging their own status, power and gaps in knowledge, especially when getting to know migrant or refugee communities.

The process of reaching towards mutual recognition is very much a two-way affair; otherwise, it will be impossible for workers to establish an identity with a community. At its most simple level, this means a worker giving local people the opportunity to see her, to put the worker in a context without feeling any obligation to begin work with her. This is close to the classic community development approach of spending a great deal of time being publicly visible, exemplified by the writing of Batten and early examples of projects: the worker deliberately walks routes in the neighbourhood that mean she passes as many groups of people as possible – people on their way to local shops, for example, or parents fetching children from school. The worker thus adds to her impression of the area, and is seen by increasing numbers of people.

The point to note about 'putting oneself about' an area is its deliberate and unhaphazard nature. For this reason, phrases sometimes used loosely by neighbourhood workers such as 'hanging about the area for a few weeks', 'wandering around' or 'getting the feel of the place' should be adopted guardedly. There are specific objectives for the worker in spending time on establishing a presence in a neighbourhood, and of course they extend beyond just the physical presence of the worker. They include, in particular, introductions and first meetings with a range of local people.

There are numerous ways by which neighbourhood workers arrive at the point of intending to work in neighbourhoods, and we do not propose to catalogue them, particularly as workers are rarely in a position to choose on their own; there will need to be discussion and negotiation with colleagues and managers. Also, a worker does not necessarily choose the most deprived of neighbourhoods within a deprived area. He or she might consider a locality which has the most community action potential in order to demonstrate what can be achieved. Resources for holding meetings, or the neighbourhood's accessibility to the worker's base, or the attitude of existing community groups could all be taken into account in making a choice.

We shall indicate the kind of action a worker is likely to take in three familiar forms of intervention: a worker assigned to work in a particular neighbourhood by her employing agency, a worker requested to work in an area by local residents, and a worker commencing work in an area as a result of a new development there, such as the launching of a government health project or the announcement of new road plans which are going to be important to local people.

Employer's mandate

It is common for regeneration teams to have no choice about the area to be worked in. A worker or team is appointed following a decision by the agency, or as a result of government policy, to place resources in a particular neighbourhood. A local authority will agree to have a project located in one part of its area of responsibility; it then has to decide in which ward the project will be placed. Similarly, a neighbourhood worker may be employed by a local authority to work, for example, on a particular housing estate; quite early on the worker will have to choose the most appropriate focus on the estate. This could be by area or by group.

When a worker is uncertain as to either the exact territory she will concentrate on out of the wider area or set of issues, a familiar technique is to help to provide information and advice services as a way of becoming established or recognised. The idea is relevant at this point because sometimes there will be services, such as information and advice, which are provided from an office in an area by a voluntary organisation or the local authority – a neighbourhood worker could also be based there for a period.

Offices of partnership agencies, local management of regeneration programmes and health centres are other examples of how negotiating entry can be facilitated in this way. An example of a neighbourhood worker obtaining a 'fast track' to being accepted and trusted by the local community came from one of the sites of an action-research project in Scotland on the connections between community development and community care. Kincardine is a large village in Fife. Despite the council having a policy commitment to community participation and decentralisation of services, it was only during the action-research process that things started to happen in this particular village. Social work staff, including a community worker, worked with community representatives to tackle not only aspects of community care planning and service delivery but also wider issues of community regeneration. Crucial to the changes were the development of a local community action team and the use of a local office as a work base for practitioners and contact point for people in the community. It provided a key starting point for the community worker who commented:

> This work has reminded me of the importance of a simple focus for community work and a non-prescriptive approach . . . to enable all potential stakeholders to get involved on their terms *not* the council's, Government, whoever!
>
> (Barr *et al.*, 2001: 17)

It is often neither feasible nor desirable for a worker to offer advice services in order to obtain a more accurate understanding of why she has been appointed to work in a particular neighbourhood and to begin to obtain a mandate from the community. The worker's chief interest at this stage will be in meeting leaders of groups and organisations. The aim will be to make herself known to them and to begin to build up a picture of the area's needs and resources, its problems and its potential. The worker will want to be aware of informal networks, in addition to established groups and organisations.

Request from local people

The context in which neighbourhood workers and other practitioners operate in the United Kingdom is complex: local authorities have to juggle with competing demands, and their agendas change constantly. This increases the possibility of a worker's role being misinterpreted – 'it has become even more important for workers to be clear and open about their roles and negotiate "agreement" and recognition of their role' (Ballantyne, personal communication). This neighbourhood worker gives the example of activists seeking community work support and yet also needing reassurance that it is not them who are to blame for the problem they wish to address.

In terms of the practitioner negotiating entry, the parameters are more obvious when a clear request has been made by local people than they are normally. This should not imply, however, a diminution of its importance of the early phase in the neighbourhood work process. However exact a request or 'contract' may be, a practitioner has always to win the confidence and trust of local people as well as become known by a range of other key actors.

Community groups and local forums can make requests for a neighbourhood worker for a number of reasons – out of anxiety as illustrated earlier, and out of despair, anger or local conflict. In her study of the Gatsby project, involving interviews with 82 groups, Liz Richardson discusses the types of help the groups received:

> Some groups credited their existence to the trigger factor of having someone there at a point they had decided to do something. A common pattern was an intensive input in the initial stages, then gradual scaling down of the high level of support as the groups became more able to operate independently. The transfer of responsibilities to the group was a delicate process, but one that groups could understand the need for.
>
> (Richardson, 2008: 211–212)

Sometimes a practitioner has run down his involvement with a group but has remained available to help it on specific issues if requested. In this case the work of gaining recognition from the group and of ensuring that the practitioner's role is clear can to all intents and purposes be short-circuited: he may simply have to renegotiate entry to the group, especially if its membership has changed significantly.

A forthright exponent of the need for the neighbourhood worker to negotiate entry only when his expertise has been requested, directly or indirectly, by local people is Alinsky (1971).

A potential issue

A commonplace characterisation of neighbourhood work is its need to be opportunistic, to 'sense the moment' at the right time. In terms of negotiating entry, two types can be identified. First, there is the practitioner who has become very well informed about, say, one local authority area, although he is not involved in neighbourhood work there. The worker has up-to-date statistics, and his contacts in different parts of the local authority structure enable him to be fully aware of future plans or of possible changes to existing plans – a decision to close a local school would be an example. The worker becomes part of several key networks, which enables him to piece together information. As a result, the worker becomes a valuable resource to community groups, because he is in a position to anticipate events and to supply crucial information.

We are referring to a strategy which arises at the local level as a result of accurate information received by a worker about a potential issue. The ticket, as it were, with which the worker goes in is prior knowledge of impending action which will affect a neighbourhood, combined with a hunch that such knowledge will be sufficient to bring about organisation within the community. The following is an example of workers using this approach to facilitate their legitimacy in a community of interest:

> Prior knowledge of impending opportunity was illustrated when, as a community development section, we noted the developing national recognition of carers and carers' issues. We recognised the extent to which carers were socially excluded as a result of their caring role and we therefore set out to develop our knowledge of carers' issues prior to negotiating entry into this community. This approach led to the development of an authority-wide carer organisation which was able to ensure that the second year of 'ring fenced' funding for carers was targeted towards carers' priorities.
>
> (Ballantyne, personal communication)

The essence of anticipating an issue seems to lie in the combination of research or investigation of facts about a community which have not been made public, along with an instinctive feel for the issue or issues which will mobilise people into some form of collective action or rekindle a dormant group. The second type of situation which opens the way for a worker can be identified as operating at more than one level. A major and complex redevelopment plan will often provide the opportunity for a neighbourhood-based regeneration team to establish itself in an area because it can demonstrate a knowledge of complex issues which threaten the future living patterns of local people. They know that good understanding of the issues, organisations and decision-making processes involved will be of vital importance in the future.

The difference between the two types of potential change is essentially that in the first case impending changes originate and take place locally, and a worker skilled at recognising early signs of planned change can communicate them to other workers and residents; in the second case, changes come from outside an area and are invariably complex and daunting for local people whom they will affect. In both cases, the worker openly makes use of his prior information to move into a position of being accepted by local people as an organiser with something important to offer. If the worker can show why it is important, he could have begun the process of winning recognition and legitimacy.

In suggesting how workers will need to draw on knowledge and skills to become recognised by existing community groups, we think that they will concentrate on meeting community leaders and influential people. Clearly they should evaluate the viewpoints of such people critically, and it will be essential later on to check out information provided by different individuals. But at this stage they are interested in achieving a broad scan of existing groups and organisations in order to obtain from them little more than an acknowledgement of their future role. There is, as yet, *no commitment to action*. Sometimes it is hard to distinguish this kind of early work from social interaction between the practitioners and community leaders, and the receptivity and hospitality of the latter will sometimes add to the blurring of the difference.

Finally, by thoughtful preparation of the way into a community, practitioners will gain an important element of confidence. As well as creating a breathing space for themselves before taking on commitments, they also know that they are laying strong foundations for later work. This is important for the inner strengths of practitioners as well as for the work itself:

> Getting started on a new job, perhaps in an unfamiliar community, is one of the most difficult – and most exciting – parts of community organising and social planning. Getting one's bearings before being thrown into the full responsibilities of a job should be a top priority for the organiser or planner beginning work in a new neighbourhood or community.
>
> (Cox *et al.*, 1977)

Getting one's bearings, finding one's way around groups, networks and community organisations, is inseparable from obtaining an initial mandate from the community.

Agencies

At the beginning of the neighbourhood work process, workers are likely to have contact with a range of agencies. However, it is vital that the number of contacts does not get in the way of the task in which we are at present interested – the need for workers to make themselves and their role known to relevant agencies, as opposed only to asking for their advice or sharing data with them. The distinction is an important one, for it is all too easy for newly arrived workers to assume either that agencies have prior knowledge of their arrival or that they understand their role. Both are assumptions that an incoming worker cannot afford to make. The need for neighbourhood workers to be more skilled at engaging with agency staff and explaining their role is a significant theme in the research carried out by Alan Barr in Strathclyde:

> For community workers to work compatibly with their colleagues they should seek common principles of operation. These should include: understanding need from the consumer perspective; recognizing and responding to both private troubles and public issues and seeing them as interconnected; seeking to liberate, not domesticate, community resources and energies; and promoting, as far as possible, a preventive approach to social problems.
>
> (Barr, 1996: 166)

It is relatively easy for an agency or coalition of agencies to undermine the future work possibilities of a neighbourhood worker before she has had time to get established and when the worker has no power base in the community to support her. The job of introducing oneself to other agencies, if it is not seen as a sensible and courteous first move, can certainly be prompted by the need to safeguard one's position. It can also be approached in a more positive spirit: as an opportunity to gain easy access to, and knowledge of, a wide range of agencies, several of which may later on be less willing to receive you so openly as on a first visit. It is politic for workers to aim to introduce themselves to a 'mix' of agency personnel: senior administrators and policy-makers as well as fieldwork staff. They should also seek to obtain a balance, in their schedule of meetings, between professional and political contacts as well as between potential allies and 'opponents'. It will often be the case that when workers are engaged in these meetings, their ability to articulate role and objectives will be most tested. Agencies such as health trusts, partnership boards, social landlords, councils for voluntary service and key departments of local authorities will usually have their own stake in the neighbourhood where a worker plans to be and will be anxious to find out about his or her intended programme and methods of work. Sometimes an agency will have a strong interest in the approach likely to be taken by a neighbourhood practitioner. A leading social landlord, for example, may appoint a director of neighbourhoods at senior management level to be responsible for the management of the agency's assets and neighbourhood teams. This person will want to hear a great deal from a neighbourhood worker coming from another agency.

The worker will need to have arguments ready. What kind of neighbourhood work – agencies may inquire – does the worker intend to do? What does the worker hope to achieve? What will the outcomes be for the neighbourhood? What will the implications of this work be for agencies? Which part of the area exactly does the worker plan to work in? These, and a host of other questions, can damage or enhance a worker's initial reputation depending on what answers are given. Some of the questions a worker will wish to answer as fully as possible, while with others – such as the exact location of the intervention – a worker will want to hold her options open.

At the same time as gleaning information from these agency contacts and explaining her role, the worker is engaged in securing explicit recognition from agencies for the work she is about to begin. At this stage, it is a transitory relationship between the worker and the agencies, whereby the worker introduces herself and thereby facilitates his or her entry into the community (later the worker may establish ongoing relationships with agencies as part of partnership working). The worker will include in her introductions other practitioners and their agencies located in or nearby the neighbourhood where she plans to work. Such meetings and observation visits will often have multi-purpose functions: other practitioners can offer an incoming worker valuable advice and information about the area as a whole, they can suggest avenues and contacts to avoid or to aim for, they can explain the kind of projects they are working on and suggest further visits, and they may offer the worker the chance of meeting some of them regularly as a support group.

The worker's agency

It may seem self-evident that making oneself known to one's own agency is an early priority for the neighbourhood worker. There will be a variety of expectations held of the worker, not only by her or his employer but also by other stakeholders – funders, partner organisations and community members. We have noted already, however, how easy it is for the task of making oneself known to be pushed to one side by the pressures to move into a neighbourhood; frequently the latter is equated in practice with an early move away from the worker's agency. Such a move is rarely deliberate: the main arena, after all, where neighbourhood work will be practised, beckons and usually the worker's own interest and motivation mean he or she needs no second asking.

A strong argument for ensuring that work is done early on with the practitioner's own agency is that of helping to guarantee self-survival: meeting those who ultimately hold responsibility for policy in the worker's agency is a necessary precaution. The worker needs to have a clear idea of the boundaries for the work perceived by the employer – even if she or he may decide to challenge them later on. Both of these points underline the importance of workers seeking, at this early stage, to obtain active and reliable support from their line managers.

Through explanatory discussions with a range of staff in the agency, practitioners can get themselves known about relatively easily and quickly. This is important in terms of role, making clear the similarities and differences between a neighbourhood work role and those of other workers in the agency. It is important also in terms of establishing future allies or contacts in the agency, in the event of the work having policy implications for the agency as a whole, or if the practitioner needs help in obtaining resources from the agency for a community group. For these reasons, a practitioner employed in a large organisation will be wise to introduce himself or herself to the relevant administrative staff as well as fieldworkers, managers and researchers.

One worker, newly appointed to a community work post with a fieldwork team of a local authority department, told us how she happened to start on a day when all the middle managers of the department were meeting:

> I was introduced to them by the chairman, and before their meeting started I went round all of them asking for their phone numbers and saying I would like to come and talk to them about their work. Most of them seemed amazed that anyone should want to do this. I saw it as a way of getting a collection of views from key staff in the agency, on how things worked and who was who.
>
> (Ballantyne, personal communication)

This may be an untypical example, and the process of a worker picking up unconnected bits of information about the agency is inevitably much longer and more haphazard. It will also, of course, vary considerably according to the type of agency in which a worker is employed. Someone joining a small neighbourhood work team in a voluntary organisation, for example, will be in a very different position from a worker located on his or her own in a large agency such as a planning or education department of a local authority. It is easier if a neighbourhood worker begins the process of introducing herself within her own agency before contacting other agencies and networks. If this work is postponed, the access is likely to be more difficult and the opportunity to attempt it may involve time-consuming negotiations later.

It is probably both sound strategy and good sense for workers to make clear early on, by the information sought and the people they wish to meet, that their work brief necessitates their working both across departments in their own agency and with a wide range of organisations at local and, occasionally, national levels. Employers of neighbourhood workers have to be aware of the need for workers to have a high degree of freedom of movement across professional and administrative boundaries, and relatively easy access, compared with most other professionals, to a range of individuals and information sources. This can include frequent and direct contact with councillors. This is particularly important given (a) widespread recognition of the idea of participatory democracy needing to complement and connect with representative democracy and (b) government policy emphasis, in England, on neighbourhood planning.

Naturally, at the same time that the worker is gaining understanding and recognition of her role among colleagues, she is also finding out useful information about the agency – about its administrative and decision-making structures, about the support a worker is likely to receive from various colleagues and sections of the agency when doing neighbourhood work, and about the likely support and cooperation she can offer them. Key questions a worker will be seeking answers to at this stage include:

- Why has this agency committed resources to neighbourhood work?
- What are the agency's assumptions about community self-determination?
- How much autonomy will the neighbourhood worker have?
- Which population groups in the community does the agency think should be served by a neighbourhood work intervention?
- Is the agency actually only interested in a specific problem area in a community?
- What resources are available to the neighbourhood worker through this agency?

Most of these points should have been covered in the job description for the worker. It is sensible, however, to check them at this stage.

Inseparable from consideration of such questions is another set of questions which focus on authority and power in the agency. To whom are workers ultimately responsible? What community interests are represented on the decision-making body – disabled people's organisations, black and minority ethnic groups, faith groups? What is the connection between the decision-making body and the funding source – identical or separate? These questions have become more relevant in recent years because of the availability of small grants for community groups through community chests and other schemes.

It is doubly important for workers to make themselves known to their agency if neighbourhood work is a new or recent introduction in the agency. Very often, in this situation, neighbourhood work has been referred to in very broad terms. It is the worker's task to sharpen up any such generalities and thereby to convey as clear an understanding of his or her role as possible. This may not mean, necessarily, that a worker should hasten to re-negotiate a job description, although that may be desirable at a later stage.

A worker's insistence on obtaining clear, agreed terms of reference for his or her work can impress upon agency colleagues the nature and purpose of the work which is about to begin in the community. The terms should be reached by the worker and the agency together. Such an educative task is continuous. It does not stop once the worker is involved in action, for the action may require the worker to influence the agreed terms. The point we are emphasising here is the wisdom of beginning the process as soon as the worker joins an agency.

We have argued that the neighbourhood worker needs to be active in three arenas in the process of negotiating entry to undertake neighbourhood work: existing community groups and organisations, voluntary and statutory agencies with an involvement in the area and the worker's own agency. The insertion of this phase at the beginning of the neighbourhood work process will prolong the total time required by the worker before beginning to form community groups; it will increase the pressures on the worker to act. It involves handling situations in the community and in agencies, as well as consideration of prior decisions and plans, before anyone is met on a more long-term basis.

Despite these real difficulties, we suggest that it is essential for practitioners to tackle the issues of acquiring information, gaining recognition, self-introduction and introducing others to which we have referred. In addition to having the functional purpose of facilitating work in the community, negotiating entry will also allow the worker time to match up impressions of the future work environment with his or her own confidence and ability.

Negotiating entry reinforces the need for reflection by workers about their own resources as workers and about the goals or vision they set themselves as they move closer to the action phase of neighbourhood work. They should now be better prepared to move into more systematic gathering of data, and we describe this in the next chapter.

References

Alinsky, S. (1971) *Rules for radicals*, New York: Random House.

Barr, A. (1996) *Practising community development. Experience in Strathclyde*, London: CDF Publications.

Barr, A., Stenhouse, C. and Henderson, P. (2001) *Caring communities. A challenge for social inclusion*, York: York Publishing Services.

Cox, F. M., Erlich, J., Rothman, J. and Tropman, J. E. (1977) *Tactics and techniques of community practice*, Itasca, IL: Peacock.

Francis, D. and Henderson, P. (1992) *Working with rural communities*, Basingstoke: Macmillan.

Jacobs, S. and Popple, K. (1994) *Community work in the 1990s*, Nottingham: Spokesman.

Perlman, R. and Gurin, A. (1972) *Community organisation and social planning*, New York: Wiley.

Richardson, L. (2008) *DIY community action. Neighbourhood problems and community self-help*, Bristol: The Policy Press.

Ross, M. (1967) *Community organisation* (2nd edn), London: Harper & Row.

Wilson, M. and Wilde, P. (2001) *Building practitioner strengths*, London: CDF.

4 Getting to know the neighbourhood

Why collect data?	How do I go about data collection?
What do I need to know?	Deciding which neighbourhood to work in
History	Taking a first look at the chosen
Environment	neighbourhood: the broad- angle scan
Residents	Some key principles in collecting and leadership
Organisations	Analysis, interpretation and write-up
Communications data	**Conclusions**
Power and leadership	

This phase of the work is variously referred to as fact-finding, data collection, assembling a community profile or audit, or carrying out an assessment of community needs and resources. The purpose of this work is to inform the practitioner's decisions about what issues, problems, groups or agencies he or she will work with. This gathering of data is rarely sufficient in itself to produce change, but is a prerequisite for planning a large number of strategies available to neighbourhood workers, other practitioners and community groups.

Fact-finding in a neighbourhood includes the following features:

- It is a specific and systematic activity which seeks to avoid haphazardness and vagueness. It is informed by purposiveness and is guided by the practitioner's objectives.
- It relates to a defined problem, issue, locality or group, and is directly concerned with the here-and-now situations of community residents.
- It is as objective and free from bias and partiality as possible in its goals, methods of collection and analysis. If it is, then workers must expect that sometimes their fact-finding will yield data that conflict with their own and others' impressions of the community.
- It is carried out with the intention of putting the findings to some use. Data gathering is not 'pure research' or the basis of a sociological study: the worker does it in order to apply its results to what she or he has to do in the community.

Why collect data?

This last point suggests one of the most important reasons why neighbourhood workers need to gather data before rushing into action. Data gathering underpins planning

DOI: 10.4324/9781003310006-4

and rationality, and simultaneously informs (and puts a limit on) the influence of intuition in the making of decisions. It is desirable that choices about what the practitioner is going to do, how it will be done and the likely consequences are based on knowledge about community groups, problems and resources. At the least, the neighbourhood worker will need to know what problems are to be identified in a community, how they are experienced by local people, and what motivation, skills and resources are to be found in the community for dealing with those problems.

There are a number of other reasons for data gathering in neighbourhood work. It provides a focused and comfortable way of initiating contacts with local people and service agencies; in respect of the latter, visits to agencies to gather facts and impressions about an area can provide the foundation for future work with those agencies and their staff. The initial fact-finding phase also provides a baseline for more specific pieces of action-research that may occur during the later phases of the life of a community group. For instance, data gathered by the worker may be useful in specific studies of, say, land ownership, employment, housing conditions and so forth that a group may need to carry out in order to support its case for particular changes in the allocation of resources. The worker's data bank on the area may also be useful to community groups when they have to prepare funding applications. While the focus of this chapter is on the gathering of information by the worker, it should not be assumed that this is solely for his or her purposes. The community should come to own and have access to most of the information.

There are various administrative issues that confirm the importance of this fact-finding phase. First, the worker has a responsibility to provide a data bank on the community that will inform his or her successors and the community. Second, it is largely through access to facts about the community that a worker's supervisor will be able to judge (a) that the worker is operating on the basis of knowledge and not guesswork or prejudice and (b) that there is a fit between the worker's interventions and his or her original assessment of needs and resources in the community. Thus, adequate data are a prerequisite of accurate monitoring and evaluation of the worker's activities, carried out by the worker and/or the supervisor. Additionally, the worker's (and supervisor's) familiarity with data about the community may often be useful in justifying and supporting some aspect of his or her work that has come under criticism. For example, a neighbourhood worker wrote an article for a local newspaper which described the very poor housing conditions in a town. Some councillors were annoyed by the article and approached the worker's manager. The worker, however, was able to show that the article was based completely on the available census data for the town.

The extent of the data gathering may range from reconnaissance studies that may take only a week or so to larger scale assessments of need that can last as long as six to nine months. Each worker must come to a decision about the scope and scale of fact-finding activities in the light of both the range and complexity of issues thought to be associated with the area, and the worker's own circumstances. A person, for example, who is an area's first worker, may have to spend considerably more time in gathering data than someone who joins a team to replace an outgoing worker. Someone who is replacing a worker will presumably have access to data already gathered and, in addition, may quickly become embroiled in action as she takes over the work left by her predecessor.

There are several other factors that will determine workers' commitments to fact-finding, including the kinds of skills they have (or don't have) for handling data, and their understanding of what they have found helpful in past experience. Likewise, the amount of time given to fact-finding will vary directly with the extent to which they see their approach as rationalist, and conversely where a worker believes in a more intuitive approach. Workers will also vary in their confidence and competence to make use of computer software packages for collecting data. There are a number of websites which give guidance on packages and on community profiling. In the rural context, village appraisals remain widely used by practitioners and local people to develop a community profile. 'Super output areas' are very relevant. They are geographical areas designed for the collection and publication of small area statistics. They are replacing electoral wards as the primary means for the dissemination of information about the local characteristics of neighbourhoods. Use of software packages can be combined with publications on community profiling such as that by Hawtin and Percy-Smith (2007).

In determining what is the 'right' balance between fact-finding and other early activities such as making relationships with residents and agency colleagues, the worker will also be influenced by an awareness of some of the 'dangers' of fact-finding. In particular, workers may be aware that gathering data can provide an inappropriate retreat from the tasks of engaging with local issues and people.

There are two questions to be asked about data collection: what do I need to know and how do I go about finding it out? The rest of the chapter is organised around these questions. Throughout, workers will need to be thinking about the extent to which they involve residents.

What do I need to know?

It is possible to specify a range of subjects about which data are sought in neighbourhood work. We have divided this range into six categories only for the purposes of analysis. In practice, they overlap and it may be difficult for the worker to know to which category a piece of information belongs. For example, data on a powerful organisation in a neighbourhood are relevant both to the category called 'organisations' and to that called 'power and leadership'. We suggest that the following scheme be used by workers as a guide or checklist in their data-gathering activities, and not as an analysis to straitjacket their own perceptions of the particular, and unique, community in which they find themselves working. In addition, some data about a neighbourhood may only make sense within an understanding of the dynamics of the whole city or region, and data about these wider areas may also be needed.

The following, then, are the six major topics about which you may want to gather data:

- History
- Environment
- Residents
- Organisations
- Communications
- Power and leadership

History

Issues and problems of an area are connected to people, organisations and events in its past. Local people are often the best sources of historical data, and contacts with them, to learn more about the history of the area, may develop to the extent that they become involved in organising around a neighbourhood issue. The need to understand neighbourhood issues within a historical perspective has generally been under-represented in the community development literature. The case for having this perspective is strengthened by the need to consider the function of a neighbourhood – whether it is settled or transitional, dormitory or 'high street', new town or outer estate – and how this connects with its history.

Environment

The environment of an area is of interest for two reasons. First, it may contain some of the problems of concern to residents (such as inadequate open space) and around which they may want to organise. Second, it provides the context in which people in the area go about their work and leisure and as such may be an important determinant of their relationships with each other.

Environmental data that are relevant for the neighbourhood worker include:

- the administrative and natural boundaries of the area;
- the density of persons per acre;
- the provision of public open space;
- the siting and effect of road, rail and pedestrian facilities;
- the volume and nature of road traffic;
- land usage in the area, and the interaction and balance between industrial, commercial and residential uses. The presence of derelict and undeveloped sites and buildings will also be something to be noted. Besides their impact on the environment, they may later prove to be a useful resource;
- the extent and nature of recreational facilities;
- the design and layout of streets and estates, and the way in which they affect residential life;
- the extent and content of residents' own creative and destructive attempts at changing the environment through activities like vandalism, graffiti, murals and fly-posting.

Residents

Data on the people who live in the area are naturally the most essential for a worker to collect. They are needed not only to understand the nature of the community in which the person is to work but also because some of this data, such as occupation and country of birth, may indicate sites of disadvantage. Data about residents may be usefully classified as follows:

Basic information

This is data about the demographic, housing, employment and general well-being of the people in the area. It includes the following information:

- **Population**. Population size and mobility, age and sex of population, country of birth, car ownership, number, size and types of households, socio-economic groups in the population, marital status, educational qualifications, morbidity/ mortality, pregnancy and other health factors and behaviours;

- **Housing**. Overcrowding, tenure, households with and without their own basic amenities like a bath, WC and hot water supply, the number of dwellings that are occupied, shared and vacant;
- **Employment**. Number of employed and unemployed by age and sex, types of jobs held by residents, numbers of men and women in part-time work, number of people travelling into and out of the area for work, and hours of work of people, especially those with children under 5 years old.

These data on population, housing and employment are obtainable from government websites and the census. One advantage of the census to the neighbourhood worker is that it provides basic data on residents for each size of area in which the worker may be interested, for example regional, borough, town and rural areas, as well as districts, wards and parishes. It must be remembered, however, that census data can often be out of date, particularly in areas undergoing major changes. Increasingly, it is being superseded as more up-to-date and accessible material becomes available.

Additional sources of data on population, housing and employment may also be available in some local authorities. For example, some of these data may be gleaned from the records of a housing department, or an authority may have carried out its own survey of housing conditions in its area.

Data on poverty

There is a potentially large amount of data that the neighbourhood worker can use to make an assessment of the social conditions of a community. Such data include free school meals, school non-attendance and exclusion, juvenile first offenders, infant mortality, electricity and gas meter disconnections, social services caseloads and referrals, homelessness and income support.

There are a number of difficulties in using such data. Much of this information is actually about the provision of services in a neighbourhood and should not be taken on its own to indicate need. Second, the ease of access to these data will vary; information on, for example, tax credits and income support is often particularly difficult to acquire.

Perceptions of the area

The neighbourhood worker will want to know residents' perceptions of the boundaries of the area, and what they see to be its good and bad characteristics as a place in which to live and work. In particular, the worker will want information on what residents perceive as the problems, issues and resources in the area, and their ideas about the causes of such problems. There will also be interest in residents' attitudes to the various sections and groups that make up the community, and towards service agencies and people like local councillors.

Community networks

Residents will be part of (or perhaps not part of) networks of relationships and contacts within their area. These networks will comprise relationships with family, neighbours and friends as well as 'nodding acquaintance' with people they recognise roam the streets and local amenities. The worker needs to understand the extent and functions of these networks, not least because they will be an important part of the support and strengths in a neighbourhood.

Community networks are also of interest to the worker because they will have an influence on his or her work in helping residents organise as a group. Such factors as the dissemination of news and gossip about an issue, the recruitment of group members and the extent to which the worker is perceived as an outsider will each be partly determined by the nature of community relationships. Neighbourhoods with a high turnover of residents will have fewer networks and connections of this sort.

Values and traditions

Adequate knowledge about values and traditions is something the worker can hope to acquire only after working in an area for a period. Yet he or she has to acquire some understanding of the diversity or nuances of community norms in the early stages of work, not least because decisions must be guided in the light of what are understood to be important values in the community. At the very least, the worker will want to avoid doing things that offend or flout conventions and values in the area. Alinsky (1971) cautioned workers to respect a neighbourhood's norms about dress, language and lifestyle. The neighbourhood worker who knowingly acts outside the standards for what is considered 'proper behaviour' in the neighbourhood risks alienating people and will be treated with suspicion, if not outright hostility.

One of the important tasks when a worker leaves a neighbourhood is to acquaint his or her successor with people's expectations about behaviour. For example, a neighbourhood worker coming new into an ongoing project described to us how:

> It has already become clear to me that there are significant 'divisions' between various estates in the neighbourhood, and that Dunstable Court is looked down upon by the rest of the blocks, even by the people in the tenements. George (the outgoing worker) warned me about the problems of using the Bull and Plough pub: he said that although it is used by Blackmills Tenants' Association, many of the people in the area think it is not a very respectable place to be in.

The kind of information the worker will be looking for in this phase of the work will largely be concerned with:

- *Norms that govern social interaction and participation in the area, particularly the neighbourhood.* For example, a worker was disappointed when few tenants turned up to a meeting in a tenant's flat. He later found out that people in the block were very circumspect about visiting each other's flats, and it was not considered 'to be the done thing'. Second, the worker who wrote about Dunstable Court tried to organise a meeting of local groups to discuss a summer playscheme. There was little interest in the meeting, largely because he had underestimated the strength of feeling against Dunstable Court; the other residents did not want to mix with them at a meeting.
- *Norms that determine people's attitudes to organising as a group and taking action to achieve some change.* Especially important are the norms that influence

the taking up and exercise of leadership and authority. Of particular interest may be the attitudes of men to the involvement of women in neighbourhood work. Neighbourhood workers continue to witness instances of male paternalism towards women and scepticism about their involvement. Women are often aware of the lack of involvement of men.

Organisations

The first difficulty that we encounter in gathering information about organisations in an area is that there are invariably a great number of them, with a diversity of goals, roles and operating procedures.

The worker must first decide on some way of conceptualising this organisational environment so as to provide a guide for the arrangement and classification of data. One way of presenting this material is simply to make a list of organisations, using a mixture of type and function to decide upon the headings for this list. This method is illustrated in the following in describing the range of organisations that the worker will seek information about.

Local and central government

This includes departments concerned with education, health, planning, regeneration, housing, employment and income maintenance. Information will be needed on each aspect of a department's work. Education, for example, will need to be looked at in terms of schools, higher, adult and community learning and youth provision. For each organisation/department, as well as various partnership bodies, the worker will seek to know:

- the nature and extent of its services;
- its structures, goals, policies, funding and staffing arrangements;
- its impact upon, and intentions for, the community;
- the nature of its relationships and communications with the community, and with other organisations;
- what resources it has that may be of use to community groups.

Economic activities

The practitioner will need to know about the production and distribution of goods and services in the community. He or she will want to know not only where people work but also the range and importance of industrial, commercial, trade and occupational activities in the area. She may try to assess the area's economic base according to whether it is, for instance, manufacturing, industrial, agricultural, commercial or recreational. She may need to construct a history and profile of major employers in the area and the extent to which industries are declining, expanding or transitional. Information about transport facilities and retail and wholesale services like shops, pubs and cafés is also useful.

Other information needed would include that on land usage and zoning and how vulnerable the area is to redevelopment, the balance between private and public industries, the character of the private rented housing stock, and the renting and management policies of its owners. The worker may want to make an assessment of:

- the long-term security and stability of the area's economy, taking into account factors such as the narrowness or breadth of its economic base;
- the relationship between the economic structure and social conditions and the nature of the community.

Faith organisations

The worker will examine these organisations to determine both what they contribute to the life of the area and the nature of any resources (such as a meeting place) they may have that would be useful to community groups. The presence and role of such organisations are often a crucial factor in trying to work with a wide range of groups and organisations in the community. These include inter-faith organisations which continue to exist in many areas despite withdrawal of funding and are crucial forums for promoting multicultural understanding and social cohesion.

Community sector

Most areas have a number of associations/groups pursuing a variety of goals with membership open to the public or certain sections of it. The minimum data that the worker will require about associations are the names and addresses of officers, and any paid staff, time and place of meetings, aims, functions and activities, numbers of members and their characteristics in terms of age, sex, class, income and residence, and an association's resources and facilities.

Voluntary sector

The worker will require similar information about voluntary organisations in the area, such as councils for voluntary service, community councils, race equality councils and organisations serving particular groups such as young people. These organisations are of particular importance to the worker because:

- they are a source of information about the area;
- they are potential participants with the worker in dealing with some community issues at a policy level;
- they are a possible target of the worker's or a community group's activities where it is seen as desirable to influence the functioning and services of the organisation;
- they are a source of resources and facilities for community groups.

Communications

It is central to the neighbourhood worker's task to understand how ideas, information and news are disseminated within the area. The worker wants to know, too, the most effective ways of communicating with key local people – whether residents or those working in service agencies. It is useful to know which instruments and channels of communication carry weight amongst particular sections of the community and help to shape and change public opinion.

The means of communication in an area will range from informal, verbal contacts on the one hand, to social networking websites, email, text messaging and newspapers on the other. The neighbourhood worker will need to study social networking websites such as Twitter and Facebook and to examine online communities dedicated to debating and discussing local issues. It will also be important to monitor websites, fly-posting, leaflets, tenants' newsletters, television and radio. As far as newspapers are concerned, the worker may find a range of products, including those of action groups, the alternative press and large circulation local newspapers. Such an analysis of media, together with contacts with individual reporters and feature writers, will help to indicate which newspapers will report sympathetically the activities of a community group.

Power and leadership

By the time the neighbourhood worker has gathered information on the residents, organisations and communications of an area, she or he will have already amassed a good deal of knowledge about how power, leadership and influence are exercised within the community, as well as across communities through cross-sectional partnerships and forums. Therefore most of the work in this aspect of data collection involves abstracting and synthesising material already gathered. We suggest that data about an area's power structure may be classified as follows:

Business and organised labour

The decisions and ambitions of the private sector and trade unions have a potent influence on the general growth and development of an area. The worker needs to understand how these two interests influence decision-making in the community, particularly that of local authority councillors and officers. Business and industry may exercise power directly, or indirectly, through organisations like a chamber of commerce or meetings of business and professional people such as the Rotary Club, Round Table and Soroptimists.

Elective politics

Here the worker will study the role and influence of political parties in the area. She or he will be interested in the strength of ward membership and the percentage of people turning out to vote at local and national elections. The worker will study the power and influence of particular ward councillors (and of the local Member of Parliament, Member of Scottish Parliament, National Assembly for Wales or Northern Ireland Assembly) and assess their contributions to policy-making at 'the town hall' and elsewhere. She or he must understand the power of the party caucus, the basis and extent of cabinet government, and the power and influence of committee chairpersons or mayor in the local authority.

Of particular interest will be the degree of involvement, if any, of the traditional political parties in working with local people on community issues. Community groups often develop to fill a vacuum created by councillors and ward parties. Groups can also be seen as unhelpful by councillors, especially in areas where one political party is dominant – the idea of a participatory democracy complementing the representative system is not accepted everywhere. In recent years, various community engagement programmes, in which there is partnership working between elected members and community representatives, have gone some way to reduce misunderstandings between the two.

Administrative politics

This phrase describes the situation where councillors have given most or all of their responsibilities for decisions to the paid officers of the council. We use the phrase also to refer to the general involvement of professional staff in organisational policy decisions. Such involvement may be accorded to staff on the basis of their professional expertise, or because staff members are given autonomy in the running of some aspects of a department's activities. It is important for the worker and groups to understand the interplay between the economic, elected and administrative personnel in an area, and their respective contributions to decision-making. In addition, the worker must identify those in an organisation who understand the nature of her or his work and would be sympathetic to the work of community groups. They may eventually provide important support and feed information to one or more groups. Many community groups fighting planning and redevelopment proposals, for instance, have been helped 'unofficially' by basic grade staff in planning departments. The policy of transparency should facilitate making data available to communities, with officials helping communities to interpret the information they get.

Civic politics

This term is used to embrace a great variety of organisations and interests who hold and influence power in a community. It includes professional, cultural and faith organisations, the media, voluntary agencies and societies, community and neighbourhood councils, advisory and management committees attached to social services and housing departments, planning forums and partnerships, and historical and conservationist societies.

Community politics

This includes groups, which consist largely of residents in the community. The groups may be organised on a geographic, identity or interest group basis. Examples are tenants' associations, residents' committees, play associations and a range of ad-hoc campaigning or action groups formed to take up some community issue or problem. Community politics also refers to meetings of groups in an area such as black and minority ethnic groups, women's groups, lodges, secret societies and cliques. We also include here the exercise of power and influence by key individuals resident in an area, who exercise their influence through an informal network of kin and social relations. The following comes from a newsletter of a busy community centre, the Sprengelhause, in the Wedding area of Berlin:

> Are you looking for a place where you can meet neighbours and eat with them, discuss a problem, or get involved with the neighourhood? A place where 'getting

older in the Sprengelkiez is just as much a topic as the encounter with and support of refugees? A gymnastics area where kita groups (under 6 year olds) romp in the morning and health sports take place in the evening? Where you can find advice or where you can help other people? The Sprengelhause is such a place.

We must stress a number of aspects of this categorisation of power and influence. First, the practitioner must be alert to the fact that alongside the formal and public power structure, there is usually a host of people attempting to influence decisions and events. These 'influentials' may range from the open campaigning of a newspaper or pressure group to the covert lobbying of decision makers by interested parties. Second, powerholders exercise that power not only in formal settings like committee meetings but also in informal ways and on informal occasions. Third, there is a good deal of interplay and overlap between the categories of power we have described. Many individuals will be involved in business as well as elective and civic politics. Finally, it would be a mistake to see power structures like a local authority or health agency as uniform and coherent systems. Any organisation may be seen to comprise individuals and groups in cooperation and conflict with each other about matters like organisational goals, policies and resources. As such, they reveal substantial tensions and rivalries that are there to be exploited by a discerning and skilful community group. It is part of the task of the practitioner to come to know these organisational 'weaknesses' and also to know to what kinds of pressures and publicity they may be vulnerable.

How do I go about data collection?

We have indicated that there is a daunting array of data that are germane to the neighbourhood worker in the initial phases of intervention. Not only must time and energy be given to choosing and gathering this data, but the worker will also be involved at this stage in other activities such as settling into the agency and making contacts with people in the community and other agencies. The multiple demands on the worker's time in this phase make it necessary that she or he comes to the task of data collection with a strategy about what data are needed and how they will be collected. Workers don't need to know everything. There is little point in workers rushing around gathering facts, figures and opinions in one hectic scramble. There are three useful questions to ask of data: Do I *need* them? What do I need them *for*? Do I need them *now*? There is the danger that without planning the worker will collect so many reports, statistics, opinions and surveys that they overwhelm his or her physical and intellectual capacity to process them. The best way to collect data is to gather them for the particular purposes at hand, rather than collecting them to store, like a squirrel, for some imagined day in the future when they might turn out to be useful.

We have found it helpful to consider four aspects in thinking about how to collect data. They are:

- deciding which neighbourhood to work in;
- taking a first look at the chosen neighbourhood: the broad-angle scan;
- some key principles in collecting data;
- analysis, interpretation and write-up.

Deciding which neighbourhood to work in

In this phase, the worker only needs data that will help decide in which neighbourhood he or she will work. In recent years, the scope for one worker to make this kind of decision has become increasingly constrained. It is likely that he or she will be a member of a team in which joint decisions are made. There will also, most probably, be clear planning and management systems in place, and these will limit the scope of a worker to make autonomous decisions. It will still be important, however, for the worker to collect comparative data and to work out the boundaries of the area in which work could be undertaken. A project, for instance, coming into a local authority will set about comparing different areas in the authority in order to choose into which area it should move. It will then need more data to decide upon a specific neighbourhood in that larger area.

In order to make or recommend this decision, the worker has to identify areas that are variously described as being in need, deprived or disadvantaged. The worker does not assume that everybody in such an area is in need but that such areas are likely to contain problems and issues which neighbourhood work could address. Thus the worker needs only those data which *indicate* likely areas of social exclusion. There are websites such as UpMyStreet (www.upmystreet.com) which provide data on a range of issues. Most large local authorities maintain websites, which include neighbourhood statistics, as do government websites such as Scotland's index of multiple deprivation. The census remains a useful source for social indicators, and our suggestion is that in this phase the worker need collect only census data that indicate a real concentration of residents who are disadvantaged in the housing, employment and education sectors. Such census data would include information on the proportion of privately rented furnished accommodation, the extent of multi-occupation and overcrowding, the existence or lack of basic housing amenities, rate of unemployment, proportion of people in semi- and unskilled occupations, and educational qualifications. Of course, if other social indicators, such as data on free school meals, are available, then the worker should also make use of them.

It must be emphasised that the choice of data from the census will be influenced by the worker's values and mandate. If his or her job is to work with particular groups in the population, such as young or older people, then the worker would obviously use the census to search for areas where such groups are to be found.

Having collected data on the different areas that are 'competing' for his or her resources, the neighbourhood worker must then rank them on each of those variables that have been taken from the census and decide which area to work in. The ranking of the areas may indicate which is in greatest need, though often the census figures may only distinguish very different areas, for example, middle-class, mainly owner-occupied districts from predominately council or housing association-owned estates. Indicators from the census will often be of limited value and will be only one of a number of factors to be considered. They will be weighed against convenience, political expediency and notions of balance and fairness. For example, a worker may decide not to work in a neighbourhood that is indicated as an area of need if, for example, there are already neighbourhood work resources to be found in it. The worker's choice between areas will also presumably be influenced by impressions formed when walking about the areas, by the views and priorities expressed by his or her agency, and by the worker's assessment of the potential for achieving change that exists in different neighbourhoods.

Taking a first look at the chosen neighbourhood: the broad-angle scan

The worker may now be ready to study the neighbourhood through what Etzioni (1967) calls a 'broad-angle scan'. The purpose of this scan is to determine the principal features of the neighbourhood and to direct the worker to those aspects of neighbourhood life and issues that he or she wishes to study in more detail. It is clearly not desirable or feasible for the worker to examine exhaustively every aspect of neighbourhood life; the worker is forced at this early stage of the work to be selective in the data collected. He or she may, of course, be selective by randomly or haphazardly choosing features of the neighbourhood to study, but we suggest that a broad-angle scan provides a more reliable and perhaps rational form of guidance as to which aspects of the community should be researched in depth. The broad-angle scan will throw up a series of:

- issues (e.g. housing, play facilities, unemployment, traffic, loneliness and neighbourhood care);
- groups (e.g. claimants, disabled, homeless and older people);
- territories (e.g. particular housing estates or streets);
- agencies, organisations and policies, or;
- existing community groups.

The worker can then decide to investigate one or more of these further. In addition, the broad-angle scan will give to the worker the 'feel' of the neighbourhood and an overview of its characteristics, both of which are essential for the collection and analysis of data about specific parts or aspects of the neighbourhood.

Before we continue, we offer some words of caution and support that should be borne in mind when reading the rest of this chapter. The emphasis and detail of our discussion of data collection may lead workers and students to spend too much time on it, or even to give up, feeling that they are not adequately prepared for the job. We have tried to be thorough and detailed in our presentation in order to provide a guide as to what *might* be done; it is not our intention to suggest that every worker should collect every kind of data to which we refer. With these words of qualification, we suggest that the broad-angle scan should comprise the following activities.

Using websites and analysing the census

The worker should use websites and the census to acquire basic information about residents of the area. As discussed earlier, the information includes age and sex, place of birth, housing tenure and conditions, socio-economic groupings, types of employment and unemployment. This will often be a re-analysis of the census data collected in phase 1.

Street work

The worker walks the streets and visits the amenities (cafés, pubs, playgrounds shops, etc.) of the neighbourhood in order to observe and talk with people. He or she must deliberately seek contact with different sections of the population and begin to understand which people frequent which parts of the neighbourhood at what times and for what purposes. Through talking with people the worker seeks indications and clues as to how people see the neighbourhood, and what they perceive as its strengths and weaknesses, issues and problems. The worker also wants to know how the people themselves divide up the area into its constituent patches – which streets go with which streets to form mini-localities within the neighbourhood.

Scanning newspapers

Find out what newspapers and magazines are read in the neighbourhood, and read through a selection of back issues. Another reading task at this stage is to obtain a preliminary grasp of the development of the area by going to the local or central library and seeing if they have a guide to or history of the neighbourhood.

Using the worker's own agency records

The worker should acquaint himself thoroughly with the records and papers of his predecessor, if any, and also scrutinise agency papers and proposals that led up to his appointment, that perhaps indicate needs and issues in the neighbourhood. Any data of his own agency on the area should be examined. Some agencies may have produced community profiles before the appointment of the worker, though it is often the case that workers are disappointed by the lack of depth in agency views of neighbourhood issues. Finally, the worker should talk with agency colleagues and understand their perceptions of the neighbourhood.

Getting to know other agencies

This includes understanding the structures and major provisions of the local authority. The worker may acquire or assemble a directory of the names and addresses of the local councillors, leading politicians, chairpersons and members of the authority's committees, and of its principal professional staff. He or she should also study the agenda and minutes from the council for, say, the past year, looking for items about the neighbourhood, and seek out reports on the neighbourhood that may have been prepared by council departments. A similar understanding of health agencies should also be undertaken.

Getting to know community groups

The worker should also get together the names and addresses of the officers of any existing community groups, and try to acquire the newsletters and minutes of these groups and begin to understand a little of their origins and functions.

Finding out who serves the neighbourhood

Here the worker wants some initial information on the range of organisations and agencies that are based in, or serve, the neighbourhood. At this stage, this kind of information may be best acquired from colleagues in the worker's agency.

Before beginning these various activities that constitute the broad-angle scan, the worker would best think about how much time and energy they will be given. When he or she has assembled and studied this information, the worker should be ready to move into the next phase, which is that of a more detailed and methodical study. However, it may often be the case that the worker feels that he has collected sufficient data through the broad-angle scan to move into the action stage of work, or the contacts the worker has made have resulted in specific requests for assistance that he feels cannot be refused or postponed. In either of these cases, the worker may decide to proceed no further with data collection. If this decision is made, the worker has to be as certain as possible that he is not moving too soon, or on the wrong issues, or with the wrong people. If, for example, the worker decides, on the basis of impressionistic conversations with people, that play is an issue in the area, he ought to be sure that play is indeed a concern in the minds of residents, and not just a 'bee in the bonnet' of those few people he talked to. One way of finding out is to 'run with an issue' and see what happens. Another way, and one which helps to diminish the possibility of an early failure marring the worker's attempts to organise within the neighbourhood, is to hold off from action for a little while longer and plan and carry out a more detailed collection of data. As workers accumulate more knowledge about a neighbourhood and consider the possible choices facing them, they need to remind themselves that the use of this knowledge is to help groups and organisations to be as effective as they can be – not simply to empower workers.

Some key principles in collecting data

Data collection should be comprehensive and detailed, and thorough and systematic in its methods. The worker wants to gather valid and reliable data rather than impressions which contribute to his or her decisions about interventions. The worker undertakes these activities by using methods and principles that reduce as far as possible the influence of chance, bias and subjectivity on his or her findings. That is, the worker attempts to provide valid and reliable data by (a) using methods of investigation that are commonly associated with social research, such as the survey, and (b) using those methods with due attention to, and understanding of, the principles that inform their use in the field of social research. For example, a worker who carries out a survey must do so with some regard to the principles of survey design and administration. There is also little value in carrying out a survey if insufficient attention has been given to matters like sampling.

The purpose of this section is only to review some of the important methods through which workers may obtain valid and reliable data. Readers must turn to specialised textbooks for further advice on the techniques and principles involved. These should include looking at less formal, more participative and collaborative methods than those presented here, for example, appreciative inquiry, storytelling or story dialogue which build on traditional, oral communication and learning techniques.

Questioning

We want to consider the two methods of questioning that seem most common and/or useful to neighbourhood workers. They are the questionnaire and focused interviews.

Questionnaires

A questionnaire may be administered by post, telephone, email or by door-knocking to deliver and collect it in person and by a face-to-face interview. Each way of administering the questionnaire, however, has its own advantages and disadvantages relating to, for example, cost and refusal rate, and the worker must assess which method is appropriate to the task in hand. On balance, the personal interview in which the worker asks the questions and records the person's responses is probably the most appropriate for neighbourhood work, not least because it brings the worker into contact with people who might later be involved in the formation of a group.

Another task for workers is to decide what *type* of questionnaire will be used. Questionnaires vary from being very standardised, on the one hand, to completely unstructured, on the other. We shall discuss the unstructured kind later in looking at the focused interview. In the standardised questionnaire, the interviewers ask the same questions in the same order to everyone who has been selected for interview. The nature of the stimulus to the respondents – the verbal questions – is kept as unvarying as possible. There are two kinds of questions on these questionnaires: the closed or 'fixed-alternative' question in which the respondents are asked to choose between alternative replies, and open questions to which the respondent may reply as he or she wishes, and the interviewer must try to record the response in full. The following are among the major issues that the worker must consider if he or she decides to become involved in surveys or self-surveys that use a questionnaire. Detailed advice on these aspects of questionnaires should be sought from a research methods textbook.

- *The design of the questionnaire.* Thought must be given to the objectives of the survey and the intentions of the worker, the issues or matters that the questionnaire must cover, the form of the questionnaire (how standardised it is to be) and the balance between open and closed questions, its length and the order of questions, and question wording. The worker must also decide how he or she will approach respondents, particularly how he or she will explain the purposes and sponsorship of the investigation.
- *Piloting the questionnaire.* It is essential to pilot the proposed questionnaire in order to 'test' it for length, relevance, wording and sequence of questions, and its overall impact on respondents.
- *Choosing a sample.* Whether or not a sample has to be chosen depends on the size of the group or population in which the worker is interested, and the time, money and help available. The advantage that sampling has over haphazardly picked-out individuals for interviewing is that it allows one to make inferences from the sample about the population from which it has been chosen.

The three kinds of sampling methods likely to be of most use to neighbourhood workers are the *simple random sample*, the *systematic sample* and the *quota sample*. In the simple random sample, each member of the population has an equal and known chance of being selected; the selection is made by assigning a number to each unit of the population from which the sample is to be drawn. Identification of the units that will make up the sample is achieved by a number of techniques, including drawing numbered discs from a bag, the use of random number tables or a computer.

Systematic sampling involves drawing every nth unit (a person or a household, for example) from a list of those units. Taking every tenth name from an electoral register, or every fifth name from a list of community groups in an area, or taking every third case from a list of an agency's clients are examples of sampling systematically. Systematic sampling is not strictly random because the people on a list do not have an equal chance of inclusion; the people who fall between the nth persons have no chance of inclusion.

In quota sampling, the interviewers are given quotas of people to interview. They are asked to interview so many people according to, for example, different age, sex, class and housing tenure groups. The number of interviews that are to be with men and women, or with different ages, is calculated from available data. For example, if 60 per cent of the residents in a street are female then the worker would ensure that 60 per cent of the people interviewed were female. The relative strengths and weaknesses of these three and other methods of sampling are discussed in specialist textbooks.

Interviewing also poses particular problems for the neighbourhood worker and for members of a community group carrying out a self-survey. On the one hand, they will be interested in building up rapport with residents; on the other, they must guard against their interests, opinions and values about neighbourhood issues influencing and distorting the replies that respondents offer.

These cautionary words about some aspects of the use of questionnaires serve to indicate that to do a survey or self-survey will require a good deal of study, time and skill. Before embarking on a survey, it is best to make sure that the information that is required is not already available, or cannot be acquired through means other than a questionnaire. The self-survey may be seen to be a more attractive proposition to the worker because it makes use of available resources in the community. But the participation of residents and/or colleagues does not necessarily represent a simple gain in numbers of people and hours. The worker will find that time has to be allocated to:

- the recruitment and encouragement of helpers;
- work with them to discuss the purposes of data collection, and the design and planning of the methods to be used;
- training them in the use of the methods if these are unfamiliar;
- supervising their work, and being available for support and discussion when helpers find problems or when their enthusiasm wanes;
- the collective analysis, interpretation and presentation of the data that have been assembled.

Additionally, there may be disadvantages to using local people or agency colleagues. Residents may be reluctant to answer questions posed by neighbours. Another argument against self-surveys is that the group which undertakes the work may too easily become the nucleus for a task or issue group that may emerge from the work carried out on the survey. People may come to expect the self-surveyors to take on the problems and the self-surveyors may not be able, or want, to handle the expectations they generate.

The self-survey has, however, advantages because of the fact that it involves local people. It is community-led. Self-surveys are more oriented to taking action on a particular issue, and are often used to prepare people for collective action by getting them involved in the collection and analysis of information. The Scottish Centre for

Community Development has published a guide on community-led action research (www.scdc.org.uk).

Focused interviews

These may be seen as less standardised and structured forms of a personal interview using a questionnaire. The interviewer has a checklist of questions or issues to raise with the respondent, who is allowed to answer them freely. Likewise, the interviewer is free to probe the respondent's replies as seems appropriate, and to add to, and modify, the interview as it proceeds if the respondent raises relevant but unanticipated issues. Such interviews are also focused by virtue of the fact that they are planned. The interviewer (in this case, the neighbourhood worker) must think about how she will present herself and her objectives, and prepare a strategy that specifies what information she wants, how to ask for it, and what factors will hinder and facilitate the interviewee's cooperativeness. The worker will need to pay attention to non-verbal communication as well as what is said, to the 'silences', for example, topics that are avoided or criticisms not articulated in words but clearly hinted at through body language.

There seem to be three primary uses to which the focused interview can be put in data collection. First, it helps the worker to understand more thoroughly how local residents perceive and describe the area in which they live. It permits the worker to acquire some understanding of how residents 'name the world'. Second, it provides the main tool for acquiring detailed information about agencies and organisations operating in the neighbourhood. Third, the focused interview is useful in acquiring more information about particularly complex aspects of community life. For example, it may be used to build up information about power, leadership and influence in a community. Additionally, the worker can interview a range of people in order to understand the different perceptions of an issue in a neighbourhood such as homelessness, unemployment or social isolation.

Before completing this section on questioning, it is worth referring briefly to a range of methods of data collection that are generally referred to as 'indirect'. They include the following:

- *Sentence completion*. For example 'If there is one change I would bring about in this neighbourhood, it would be . . .'
- *The projective question*. For example 'Suppose a Person from Mars came down to this neighbourhood, and you were the first person she saw, and she asked you what kind of neighbourhood this was; what would you tell her?' Another form of the projective question involves asking the respondent about the views of other people, for example 'Some people who live in this estate find a lot of faults with it. I wonder if you can guess what they are referring to?'
- *Adjective checklist*. Respondents are shown a list of varied adjectives that purport to describe the neighbourhood. The respondents are asked to say which they think apply.
- *Inventories*. There are two kinds which seem potentially useful in neighbourhood work. With the first, respondents are shown a list of problems/needs and asked to indicate the problem(s) that most affect them as residents in the neighbourhood.

The second kind of inventory contains a list of general statements (e.g. 'Shopping facilities for older people in this area are poor'), and respondents are asked to say whether they are true or false or indicate on a scale the extent to which they agree or disagree.

Indirect methods such as these originated in clinical and social psychology but are now used in community settings, not least by market researchers. We believe they offer a useful alternative to questionnaires for the neighbourhood worker engaged in data collection.

Observation

By this phase of intervention, observing what goes on in the neighbourhood will have become second nature to most workers. But observation can be undertaken in a more systematic fashion, paying more regard to certain principles and care in the collection, recording and analysis of the data obtained. In order for it to result in useful, reliable data, it is important that the neighbourhood worker spends time on these organisational aspects.

One of the first decisions for the worker wishing to organise a more systematic form of observation is the degree of participation. At one extreme, the worker can be a complete observer with very little interaction with the observed, who may not know what the worker is or what her job in the community is; at the other extreme, the worker will be so keen on building up relationships with local residents that she maximises participation and attempts to share as many experiences of the observed as possible. This stance may endanger objectivity. As with personal interviews, the worker must strike a balance between satisfying her requirements as a neighbourhood worker and satisfying those as an investigator and a collector of information.

One thing is clear, however; the worker will seldom want to be a totally passive observer. It will be found that the degree of participation with those being observed will vary with factors like the time the worker has been in the neighbourhood and the social setting in which the observations are taking place. A more active role is also made likely by the fact that participant observation consists not only of observations but also of questions of, and interviews with, those being observed. The participant observer's use of questioning is, of course, in accord with the values and principles of questions within neighbourhood work practice. It underlines the value of the practitioner constantly posing the question why. Why are these things being said? Why is it difficult to obtain answers to such and such a question?

There are two types of questioning that seem to be part of the participant observer's techniques for gaining data. They have been described by Strauss *et al.* (1964) as the *reportorial* type of question in which respondents are asked informally about the who, what, where, how and why of events, and the *posing* types of questions. Strauss distinguishes between the following types of posing questions:

* *The challenge or devil's advocate question.* The fieldworker deliberately confronts the respondent with the arguments of opponents. The idea is to elicit rhetorical assertion and thus to round out the respondent's position by forcing him to respond to challenge.

- *The hypothetical question.* This kind of question is another technique for rounding out the respondent's thought structure but without accompanying rhetorical heat. The fieldworker poses a number of possible occurrences (e.g. 'What would happen if you stopped paying rent?').
- *Posing the ideal.* There are two variations on this technique. First, the respondent can be asked to describe the ideal situation. Secondly, while the fieldworker can still pretend to be somewhat naive, he can assert an ideal to see what response is elicited. Happily, what usually happens is that, when the investigator poses an ideal, respondents not only counter with other ideals, but also, in the process, tend to point out the shortcomings of reality.
- *Offering interpretations or testing propositions on respondents.* It is sometimes very useful to tell respondents about the propositions that one is beginning to pull together about events interesting to them. If they disagree, they will usually volunteer information to counter a proposition, which may lead the fieldworker into further unanticipated search. If they agree, the tendency is to qualify the proposition: it does not quite meet the case. Again, the fieldworker comes away with additional valuable information.

(Taken in full from Strauss *et al.*, 1964,
and reprinted in McCall and Simmons, 1969)

As with other forms of collection, attention has to be paid in participant observation to the design of fieldwork, sampling, entering the fieldwork situation, record-keeping, and the interpretation and analysis of data. Recording observations is particularly difficult in participant observation, and most observers have to rely on a combination of memory, symbols and discreetly written notes.

Using written materials

We have already stressed that websites and the census are likely to prove the most valuable written source of data and we have already indicated what data should be extracted from them in the broad-angle scan. In this section we wish to deal briefly with three other types of written material.

Local newspapers

A worker in a neighbourhood may want to undertake a more systematic analysis of the content of local newspapers in order to add to knowledge of felt and expressed needs.

The special technique for analysing the content of the media is called *content analysis*. The first task is to decide which local newspapers to study. It is fortunate that most neighbourhoods are served by only one, at the most two, large circulation local newspapers, so the worker may decide to study all the local papers read in the neighbourhood. These papers are also likely to be weeklies. The worker may also decide to study the content of newsletters and community newspapers put out by community groups.

It is unlikely that time will be available to study all the issues of local publications, so the worker must prepare a *time sample*. He or she might, for instance, decide to study all the issues of the local weekly newspaper that have appeared in the last six months, that is, about 26. How many issues to read and analyse will partly be determined by how much time is available, and the worker can clearly choose a larger sample if help is available from local people or colleagues. The next step is to determine which parts of the newspaper will be studied – headlines, editorials, features, news, photographs and so on. Alternatively, the worker may decide to analyse the content of the whole of the newspaper.

The most basic aspect of content analysis is to note the frequency with which certain items appear in the newspapers. So the worker must decide what kinds of items are to be counted. For instance, he or she may prepare a list of categories of need or issues in the neighbourhood such as play, housing, transport and shopping facilities. The worker will need to be clear what the 'rules' are for classifying an item within one of these categories. He or she then proceeds methodically to classify newspaper items within these categories, noting the number of appearances of articles, features, editorials, letters and so on, concerned with one of the categories. When this has been done, the worker is in a position to count up the items found in the categories, and this will give a simple quantitative indication of which issue seems most important to the press (as measured by the frequency of its appearance).

Counting the number of times an issue appears is, of course, a superficial form of content analysis. A worker who wants to improve on this can use refinements like considering the amount of space that is given to various neighbourhood issues by measuring column inches. The findings of a content analysis such as the one described are not unambiguous. The frequency with which issues are mentioned may just as well reflect the editorial policy, or interest of the paper, as felt and expressed needs in the community. The usefulness of data derived from a content analysis of papers is that they can be added to the worker's store of knowledge about the neighbourhood that has been acquired from a range of other sources.

Local history sources

Having gained some familiarity with the area's history, the worker may now want to extend and deepen this knowledge. The best way to start doing this may be to go to the local or central library which will contain books, guides, directories and maps about the neighbourhood and its hinterland. It may also possess primary source material like archives and public, family and business records. There will almost certainly be a librarian who will not only advise on primary and secondary sources but may also be a source of information in his or her own right. Some libraries also produce written guides to available local history sources. Another useful place to seek information and advice is a local history or civic society.

Most workers will have limited time and interest in understanding the local history so presumably they will need to be selective in what they study. A worker, for instance, might only want to know about the development of a particular trade or industry or geographical patch, and this will provide the boundaries for the inquiries. Some may choose to get an all-round appreciation of the neighbourhood's history. In this case, they might confine their study to getting information on the origin and growth of the settlement, changes in population size and structure, housing and living conditions, the economics, occupations and employment of the neighbourhood, and changes in values and traditions, particularly as they relate to socialisation processes through institutions like the family, education and religion.

Any worker who believes it is important to study primary sources of information needs to be aware that there are, as in all other aspects of data collection, systematic and thorough ways of proceeding.

Agency records

The worker will have examined his or her own agency's records, and will also have used information from a variety of agencies in compiling the social indicators that were used to help in the decision about which neighbourhood to work in. Data from agency records also complement the profiles on agencies' structures, services and policies that the worker constructs from focused interviews with agency staff.

The neighbourhood worker may make a special study of agency records, not just to gain additional information about the agency, but also largely to understand more about needs and issues in the neighbourhood. Most central and local government agencies gather data about their service users quite routinely. Such data include, for example, social services case record analyses, health and education statistics, and crime records. Besides records on their services and users, most agencies also produce reports, minutes, brochures and annual reports.

There are difficulties in using agency data. The geographical areas for which local agencies keep data are seldom coterminous, and often they are larger than the area or neighbourhood in which the worker is interested. In such cases, the worker may need to seek access to the raw data from which the agency's records have been compiled – confidentiality and data protection permitting.

Analysis, interpretation and write-up

It is misleading to present analysis, interpretation and write-up as terminal activities in the fourth phase of data collection. They are, and ought to be, ongoing activities to which the neighbourhood worker pays attention from the first phase of data collection. Analysis of data must go hand-in-hand with its collection, if only to guide the worker in decisions about further material required. Each phase of the process of data collection should end with a review of the data so far assembled so that they may inform what has to be done in succeeding phases. It is also more efficient, interesting and less error-prone to analyse and write up data as one proceeds, rather than leaving oneself with a large amount of information to wade through at the end of the process of collection. Analysis and interpretation of quantitative and qualitative data about a local neighbourhood demand of the workers' skills and objectivity of a high order.

There are two major aspects of the analysis and interpretation of neighbourhood data. First, the data must be scrutinised in relation to their validity, reliability and relevance. The worker has to decide which data ought to be put aside, which should not be used because of data protection legislation and which may be safely and honestly used as a basis for decisions about work. The claims of conflicting or contradictory pieces of information have to be evaluated. Second, the data have to be 'broken up' in order to discern the various issues, trends and relationships that they contain. While the highest possible standards of analysis have to be brought to bear on the data, it is equally important that the worker does not lose sight of the fact that the collection and analysis of data have been undertaken as an aid to action. They must thus be analysed and written up in ways that facilitate decisions that the worker must take about future activities.

Writing up the data

The extent and nature of the report of the data will largely be determined by what the worker plans to do with the report. Writing up one's analysis and conclusions is only part of a total process, and the worker must decide what his or her objectives are in spending time and energy on writing a report. What the worker intends to do with the report, or the kind of action he or she envisages taking when the report has been produced, should determine the kind of report written.

Report writing, like most things, ought to be planned, and one of the key planning questions is: for whom will I be writing this report of my data collection? In other words, who will be the kinds of people to read it? You might expect that the write-up will be read by as diverse an audience as community residents, agency colleagues and managers, elected members and staff in other agencies concerned with the neighbourhood. If this is the case, then the worker must consider two further issues in planning a report:

- *Is one report sufficient?* Should I not consider writing a number of reports, each one geared to a particular set of readers? The worker might consider that a report that is suitable, say, for his or her agency may not be the most appropriate for influencing councillors or for raising awareness among residents about the needs and issues 'uncovered' in the collection of data.
- *How do I empathise with my potential readers?* In order to make an impact with the report, the worker must think herself into the minds of those for whom she or he is writing, trying to assess the kind of write-up that best communicates to them. It is worth spending time thinking what would be the most effective means of getting the attention of particular target groups of people. Thus, a computer laptop or video footage presentation may be a more appropriate medium for local people (and councillors?) than a written report. It is crucial that the language used is appropriate for the people to whom the communication is directed, ensuring that the ideas and concepts are clear and convincing the audience that what they read is relevant to their needs and purposes. Saul Alinsky has summarised all these prescriptions for effective communication in the phrase 'always communicate within the experience of your audience'.

Besides recognising that there may be a need for varying the medium, style and content of the write-up for each target group, there is also the fact that the communication of the products of the data collection may be achieved through different *types* of report. These include the following types:

A data bank: This will comprise the raw material gathered by the worker, including quantitative data and the results of observations, focused interviews and content analyses. These data may have to be consulted by the worker, and other staff and residents, in the future, in order, for instance, to make a funding application. Again, the issues of confidentiality and data protection will need to be considered.

Working papers: Another possibility is to write papers around each of the major issues or themes that have emerged in collecting data. The worker, for instance, might want to prepare a paper on homelessness, income maintenance or about a particular estate or set of streets.

Feedback papers: Papers might be prepared that provide feedback to those from whom the worker received information or who helped in the collection of data. The feedback might be about the outcomes of the data collection as a whole, or about the specific interests, services and so on, of those interviewed.

Popular papers: These might include articles for newspapers, websites, tenants' newsletters, broadsheets and leaflets that help to disseminate the findings of the data collection to a wider and lay audience.

Organisation profiles: In the course of their data collection, much information would have been collected about serving the neighbourhood. This material can be brought together in the form of profiles of the most important organisations, and these may be useful to the worker and community groups in future relations with the organisations.

Survey reports: There may be a case for separate reporting of any surveys that have been undertaken during the collection of data, for example, surveys on the needs of older and disabled people. It may be advisable to deal with these separately because they may be suitable for a distribution that is wider than the neighbourhood or even the particular local authority.

Community profile: This is the report in which the worker seeks to present data about the neighbourhood as a whole. It may take one of two forms. First, a limited neighbourhood analysis. This is a selective presentation of the data, and the selection is made on the basis of some of the decisions the worker has already made about what his or her future activities are likely to be. It presents the data that provide evidence either for the worker's preferred analysis of issues in the neighbourhood or for decisions taken about possible action. The second form of community profile is more comprehensive. It seeks to bring together in an ordered manner all of the data that the worker has gleaned about the neighbourhood. As such, it may also be widely used as a source of data, together with the data bank of the raw material.

We do not suggest that it is necessary for every neighbourhood worker to prepare all of these kinds of report of data collection. To do so would be to give to data collection a proportion of field time that may not be justified. The point is that workers are aware that there are a variety of forms of writing up their data and disseminating it, and they should choose those that seem most appropriate in the light of the data and the worker's own circumstances. Nor do we want to suggest that the writing up of data will come to an end at the termination of data collection. There will be many occasions when both workers and groups will need to refer to the data and write it up for some special purpose. In particular, the data are likely to be used to support applications for funds and other resources. The writing of funding proposals, whether to one's own authority, central government or trusts, is a skilled activity in its own right, about which neighbourhood workers and groups should seek advice before switching on the computer.

Conclusions

While this chapter has been concerned with the collection of a wide variety of data about a neighbourhood, it has tended to emphasise the collection of data that indicate the existence and extent of issues and problems. But the worker will also be collecting information about the resources and strengths of an area, and assessment of these must also feature in a written analysis of the data he or she has collected. Doing a SWOT analysis (strengths, weaknesses, opportunities, threats) can be a useful way of ensuring that there is a balance between apparently negative and positive features of a neighbourhood. The worker can do the analysis on his or her own or with residents and colleagues. Neighbourhood workers have also used several different methods of classifying information about resources and making it available to groups and to agency colleagues. These include plotting resources on maps and the use of resource directories.

There are two other important activities that neighbourhood workers are involved in simultaneously with data collection: making contacts with local people and developing working relations with colleagues and managers in their own agency. Both activities can lead to early requests for help, or the involvement of the worker in agency activities such as membership of an agency working party. Workers have thus to manage their time and commitment in data collection in relation to these other demands made upon them. Additionally, the phases of data collection and making contacts are frequently described by neighbourhood workers as amongst the most stressful and lonely in the whole process of neighbourhood work.

We end this chapter by repeating a point we have made several times before: data collection is not a research project to be pursued for its own sake. It is done in order to facilitate planning and action. Data collection, analysis, planning and action are the key and inter-locking ingredients of a systematic approach in neighbourhood work. At the end of data collection, the worker should be able to prepare an options paper that specifies the actions that might be taken in the light of identified issues and resources. The preparation of a plan of intervention is the subject of the next chapter.

References

Alinsky, S. (1971) *Rules for radicals*, New York: Random House.

Etzioni, A. (1967) 'Mixed-scanning: a "third" approach to decision-making', *Public Administration Review*, 1; also in N. Gilbert and H. Specht (1977) *Planning for social welfare*, Englewood Cliffs, NJ: Prentice-Hall.

Hawtin, M. and Percy Smith, J. (2007) *Community profiling. A practical guide* (2nd edn), Maidenhead: Open University Press.

McCall, G. J. and Simmons, J. L. (1969) *Issues in participant observation*, Reading, MA: Addison-Wesley.

Strauss, A., Schatzman, L., Bucher, R., Ehrlich, D. and Sabshin, M. (1964) *Psychiatric ideologies and institutions*, New York: Free Press.

5   What next? Needs, goals and roles

Assessing the nature of problems and issues	Setting goals and priorities
Description of the problem	Deciding on role disposition
Definition of the problem	Factors that affect role
The extent of the problem	Role choice and role arenas
The origins and dynamic of the problem	Specifying the next moves
Recognition of action about the problem	Summary

Planning is a purposeful and conscious act of anticipation through which we attempt to envisage the future. Through planning we seek to attain future states seen as desirable and to avoid those that we see as undesirable. Planning may also be used to keep things as they are. It is through planning our activities that we try to reduce our reliance on chance and accidents in attaining our goals. In this way, we plan in order to bring more certainty and predictability to our future activities and, in addition, to make them more certain and predictable to those who work with us. It is through planning, too, that we are able to state goals and targets and be in a position to monitor progress in achieving those goals.

Thinking about things in our heads before we rush into action does not mean that workers should, or will be able to, stick rigidly to plans once they have been conceived. Workers must be prepared, first, to modify their intentions in the light of changing circumstances in the community and in the organisations and groups that affect their work and, secondly, be alert to chance events in the turbulence within and around a community group.

We suggest that there are four major tasks for the worker to accomplish in deciding what to do next. They are:

- assessing the nature of problems and issues;
- setting goals and priorities;
- deciding on role expectations;
- specifying the next moves.

We shall look at each of these in turn.

Assessing the nature of problems and issues

As a result of collecting and assessing data, the worker will be aware of those factors in the neighbourhood that are seen by residents and professionals (and by the

DOI: 10.4324/9781003310006-5

worker) as concerns, issues or problems. Undertaking these tasks would have helped the worker to discover the issues of greatest salience for people. In effect, the worker will draw up a list of such problems and issues – unemployment, play space, people who are house-bound, bad housing and environment, poor health, lack of trust between adults and young people, inadequate shopping facilities and so on – and a next step will be better to understand these issues through a *problem analysis*. We use this term with caution as we do not wish to imply that there are not opportunities, hopes and assets in communities. 'Problem analysis' is about responding to situations of potential change, about setting out the nature and scale of a problem as a prelude to working with local people on it.

Such an analysis requires the worker to define the problem or issue and spell out its key dimensions, to understand how the problem is defined and labelled (e.g. by residents and elected members), to determine the size and scope of the problem and to gather evidence, theories and hypotheses that might help to explain the causes and persistence of the problem.

The assessment and analysis of problems and issues may, for the purposes of discussing them here, be separated out into the following major components.

Description of the problem

The worker's first task in problem analysis is to try to understand how the issues that have been 'discovered' are described by the variety of people with whom he or she has been in contact. We suggest here that descriptions of problems are different from definitions of problems (to be discussed next) and the worker must try to understand the ideas, concepts, words, phrases and so on that people use in their everyday descriptions of the problem. In particular, the worker must attend to the everyday descriptions that local residents use, and be alert to the content and nuances of the vocabularies in the neighbourhood used to 'name the world' and its problematic features. Building up knowledge of these descriptions is part of the continuing process of increasing one's familiarity with a neighbourhood and identification with its inhabitants. There are three important reasons why the neighbourhood worker should attune himself to people's problem descriptions.

First, the worker is more likely to stay within people's experience if he is familiar with the way in which they are accustomed to think about and describe problems that they face. Alinsky (1971) has also pointed out that familiarity with people's experience 'not only serves communication but also strengthens the personal identification of the organiser with others, and facilitates further communication'.

Second, the worker needs to empathise with local people, to put himself in their shoes, and try to understand the problems as they experience them. Such empathising is a sound counter-weight to any inclination on the part of the worker to 'intellectualise' residents' problems, or to attribute to them perceptions of a problem that are largely his own.

Third, the language that residents use to describe problems may provide an indication to the worker of their motivation to do something about those problems. Language can be a significant clue both to the extent to which people are critically reflecting on the problematic features of their situation, and of the degree to which people feel able enough to challenge the forces that they see as creating those problems. Descriptive language thus points to the inner political world of community residents, and may be suggestive of the extent of the feelings of powerlessness, alienation, resignation and apathy, as well as feelings of hope and determination.

Definition of the problem

The worker's task here is to extend his or her understanding of the key historical and operational dimensions of the problem or problems. While a major question in approaching the first stage of *describing the problem* is how do people *experience* this problem?, the question now is 'how is this state of affairs described by residents, *defined* as a problem, by whom, and why?'

We have here introduced the distinction between a state of affairs or a situation and a problem. This distinction is important because people may describe a state of affairs (such as 'My flat has no central heating') without also perceiving and defining it as a problem. States of affairs become problems only through a process of definition and labelling (usually because the states of affairs threaten important local or national values). The worker must not assume that because states of affairs in the neighbourhood are defined as problematic by himself and other professionals, they are necessarily seen as such by residents. A worker may be appalled by the housing conditions in a tower block and also puzzled that tenants do not define the conditions as problematic. The tenants may be aware primarily only of the advantages of their flats (e.g. cheap, centre-city living), or they may be resigned to low expectations and have few ambitions about their housing rights and conditions. In this latter situation, of course, the neighbourhood worker may find that a prerequisite of organising tenants around the issue of their housing is that she first raises the level of their consciousness about their situation.

Thus, the worker wants to know, first, do residents define states of affairs as problematic? If so, how and why are they so defined? Second, if these states of affairs are defined as problematic in the wider society, what are the key historical, conceptual and operational features of the problem definitions? As far as the historical and conceptual features are concerned, the worker who, for example, is working with the problem of housing, will want to understand better what 'over-crowding' and other key concepts mean. A worker alerted to the problems described by, say, mothers in a tower block will want to know what 'isolation' or 'safety' means. The operational features of a problem would include analysis of the laws and conventions relating to the problem and the administrative/political structures in which decisions in respect of the problem are taken.

The worker may not, of course, have the knowledge or the previous experience to be able to explore the definitions of all the problems encountered. No one person can be expected to be competent in all aspects of the diversity of problems generated in inner-city areas in the fields, for example, of housing, public health, employment, welfare rights, transport, planning and education. Most workers will have to 'mug up' on problems as they are thrown up by the community – this is where high-quality professional development supervision, as compared with managerial supervision, is important, especially in helping the worker find appropriate experts to discuss the particular problem area.

There are, of course, limits to the thoroughness with which the worker can explore the definitions of the particular problem. Limits are set by scarcity of time and energy, the absence of available or understandable expert opinion and the pressing need for action on the problem or issue.

The extent of the problem

An analysis of a problem would be incomplete without an understanding of its size, scope and effects, and the following seem to be the primary points for consideration:

- What are the numbers of people affected by the problem? How many are affected directly, and how many are affected indirectly or peripherally? To what extent is the problem a public issue rather than a private trouble?
- In what ways does the problem affect the people involved? How does it influence and determine the various aspects of their lives?
- How long has this situation lasted, and how long has it been experienced as a problem by the people? For how long will it persist if the people do not do something about it themselves?
- What is the geographical locus of the problem, that is, in which parts of the neighbourhood/estate/block, etc. is the problem to be found?
- What social values are threatened by the existence of the problem (and led to a state of affairs being labelled as problematic) and which values and norms in the neighbourhood support, and which oppose, the existence of the problem or problems; that is, which individuals and sections of the community stand to gain, and which stand to lose, by attempts to ameliorate or eliminate the problem?

Arriving at an idea of the extent of a problem, however, is not just a matter of aggregating quantitative data; it also involves assessing qualitative data about how people experience the problem.

The origins and dynamic of the problem

Having defined the nature and extent of the problem, the worker will need also to understand how that problem has come about, to ask questions about its origins, and to think about factors that he or she believes are responsible for causing, perpetuating and aggravating the problem. In other words, the worker will have hypotheses about causation that are an integral element of problem assessment because they will presumably have an important bearing on the kinds of 'solutions' the worker will come up with.

The relationship between a worker's causative theories and the subsequent interventions she makes is not, however, necessarily logical and consistent. For example, a neighbourhood worker may believe that the poor housing of the tenants was brought about by structurally determined inequities in the ownership, distribution and consumption of income, wealth and other resources. But her mode of intervention with the tenants may be more or less the same as that of another worker who holds a different view about the causes of poor housing, who thinks that poor housing is an unfortunate problem in a private and public housing market that on the whole operates to everyone's benefit. Both workers, with different theories of causation, might nevertheless intervene to organise the tenants into a group and help it develop an action plan.

There are, of course, other situations in which the neighbourhood worker's theories of causation will determine her interventions and distinguish them from those that another worker might make in the same situation. For example, local people might see their major problem as vandalism and delinquency in the neighbourhood. One worker might say the 'cause' of the vandalism was associated with the poor housing conditions, while another worker would say it was caused by lack of recreational opportunities. The first worker would organise a tenants' housing action group, and the second worker might run a summer playscheme with a committee of interested parents. In this case, their interventions are different and follow from their individual causative theories. The first worker might also want to draw the group's attention to the relationship between their 'local' problem and those factors that he or she believes cause and shape the problem at city-wide, regional and national levels. Certainly, the nature of a worker's causative theories will determine the extent to which he or she is willing and able to set neighbourhood issues within a broader political and administrative context.

Recognition of action about the problem

The tasks of problem assessment might conclude with the worker setting down what has been discovered about people's readiness in the neighbourhood to take action in respect of the problem(s) they have mentioned. Besides *readiness* for action, the worker also needs to know what action various people think will be *effective*, and what they will *contribute* to that action by way of time, commitment, skills, resources and so forth. There are thus three practice questions for the worker:

- Are there any people who are ready to act?
- If so, how do they want to act, and under what conditions will they be prepared to act?
- What are they willing to contribute to the action?

Similar questions are suggested in the LEAP framework discussed in Chapter 2:

- Motivation – what may stimulate people to address a need or problem?
- Capacity – have they the resources needed to support the action?
- Opportunity – what situations are available to trigger and focus action?

(www.scdc.org.uk)

In order to ask and answer these questions, the worker will need to differentiate between the various actors in the neighbourhood so far encountered. In particular, the worker will need to be clear about:

- the service agencies and other organisations who have shown an interest in respect of the problem(s);
- existing groups of residents who have expressed concern about the problem(s);
- any individuals who have said they would be willing to help;
- the conditions under which they will help.

The clarification of this information by the worker has two purposes: first, it provides some preliminary data on residents that will have to be considered in thinking about the feasibility of particular goals and strategies; second, it helps to prepare for his or her work in more systematically contacting groups and individuals with a view to organising them for neighbourhood action of one kind or another.

Setting goals and priorities

The next phase in working out what to do next is for the worker to clarify his or her own goals and priorities and those of the employing agency. The necessity for considering goals and priorities is based on the assumption that, in most neighbourhoods, the worker will be faced with responding to more needs and demands than there is the time, energy and resources to meet. Personal goal setting as a way of making a considered choice between the bits of work that might be taken up does not imply pre-empting or encroaching upon the decisions that local groups and people have to make about their goals. Nor is personal goal setting inimical to a worker operating non-directively because this goal setting precedes the worker's real engagement with local people and groups.

On the other hand, such personal goal setting by the worker may unwittingly *influence* those decisions that local people have to make. One cannot assume that any issue has as much chance as any other in being thrown up by the community. In practice, the knowledge and skills of its worker will have some influence, even without him or her wishing it, on the judgement of local people about what issues can viably be pursued.

Setting goals and priorities is largely concerned with:

- choosing which of several 'competing' neighbourhoods or small geographical territories to focus on in respect of the problems and issues previously identified;
- choosing which of a number of existing groups and organisations to work with, if any, and/or deciding what help to give to establishing new residents' organisations;
- deciding whether to respond to the overtures and demands for help that will have by this stage come from agencies in the community;
- deciding how to respond to the demands made by one's own agency. Here the worker has to decide how much of the work will be focused on the neighbourhood and how much on fostering change and development within his or her own agency;
- deciding which of the identified problems/issues the worker will choose to pursue. This may involve consideration of the balance between 'quick wins' and longer term struggles.

This last area of choice has two dimensions. First, the worker is likely to have identified a number of problems, most of which have salience for the people in the neighbourhood. She has to decide, in consultation with local people, groups and her own agency, which of these problem areas will be pursued; that is, the worker has to establish some priority among these problem areas. In addition, the worker needs to take the following factors into account:

1 The mandate and resources within the agency for pursuing the various problem areas. It may well be that a worker will have to give little or no priority to problems with which she or he and the agency have no mandate and authority to deal

and in this kind of case the worker's task may be to 'refer' the problem to workers in another agency who do have the appropriate mandate to intervene.

2   Deciding on goals and priorities in the light of the worker's own experience and skills. Does she or he have the right experience and skills to help people in respect of a particular problem?

3   The worker's own values and preferences are an important element in establishing priorities, and choices made on the basis of the worker's values may conflict with choices suggested by agency-determined priorities, or by felt needs in the community.

The second dimension of choice about problems is that of refining banner statements of goals (there is a further discussion of goal setting in Chapter 8) to statements about sub-goals, or options towards the overall goal, and the ways in which they will be achieved. The sub-goals will represent an initial specification of the activities and strategies the worker will use in order to achieve major goals. For example, the worker might have chosen as a priority to 'run with' the issue of inadequate play facilities in the neighbourhood. The worker's banner goal statement might then read: 'to work on improving play facilities for X age group'. Some of the sub-goals that may be consequent on this major goal are shown in Figure 5.1.

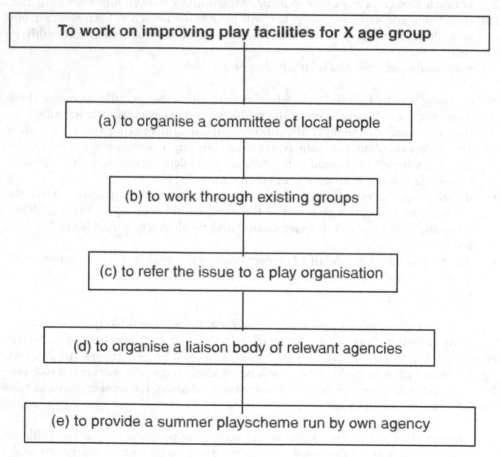

Figure 5.1 An example of banner and sub-goals

The sub-goals are in effect instrumental goals through which the larger goal of improving play facilities may be achieved. The sub-goals specify the objectives for the worker, and as such they predict the range of roles and activities from which the worker can choose in order to achieve his or her particular objectives. The worker needs to be aware of the criteria to be used to decide upon which sub-goals to pursue. Such criteria include the following:

1   Is the worker interested primarily in process or product results? That is, does she give priority to the learning goals that local people achieve through neighbourhood action, or is she more concerned to get tangible end products into the neighbourhood? A worker interested in process goals will clearly choose sub-goals (a) and (b) in this particular case, whereas a worker who thinks it more important to get a play resource into the area may choose sub-goals (d) and (e) if she believes that working through agencies will produce the resources more quickly.
2   How urgent is the need for an improvement in play facilities? A worker who is caught up in a crisis about vandalism and delinquency may feel the pressure to provide an immediate playscheme, organised by herself and staffed with 'professional' workers, and only then feel able to move into organising local people around the issue of play.
3   Which of the sub-goals is the worker best equipped to work on in terms of time, energy, skills and experience?
4   What constraints and opportunities attach to the worker's mandate, role and status, and to those of her agency, that seem to suggest that some sub-goals may be more feasible than others? It sometimes happens that a worker will be influenced in choice of sub-goals by considering which are likely to be quickly achieved. This is often brought about by pressure from the worker's agency to produce results. Acting in this way can also help the worker establish credibility within a neighbourhood.

Deciding on the nature of the role

Let us assume that the neighbourhood worker has to work at the task of getting people organised around the specific issues/problems that have been identified in the neighbourhood. The worker must not only think about making contact with local people (see Chapter 6) but must also consider the kind of role she is predisposed to play in her transactions with local people. We use the term 'predisposed' because we do not believe that workers should stick to a role or roles without regard to the situation in which they and the group find themselves. Sensitivity and flexibility are the key words to ensure that the neighbourhood worker adopts roles that will push forward, rather than hinder, the work of the neighbourhood group.

There is a proliferation of labels in community work literature that describe the roles open to the worker. 'Interpreter', 'communicator', 'enabler', 'guide', 'facilitator', 'encourager', 'catalyst', 'broker' and 'mediator' are labels that may be taken to suggest objective, neutral, democratic and even laissez-faire roles on the part of the worker; other words like 'stimulator', 'expeditor', 'organiser', 'negotiator', 'bargainer', 'advocate', 'expert' and 'activist' suggest more active or directive roles for the neighbourhood worker.

The abundance of labels may confuse the practitioner who is intent on choosing the role(s) that seem most appropriate. The worker may be confused, first, because the proliferation of labels has not been fully matched by attempts to define the activities associated with them; second, she will find little consensus in the literature about either the extent of the range of possible roles, the definitions of such roles, or their desirability or likely effectiveness; and, third, the elucidation of roles in the community work literature sometimes conveys the impression that the worker's choice is an all-or-nothing commitment to one role and a rejection of the others. We believe that the worker's choice of role should be either a tactical or strategic decision, and that workers will move in and out of different roles according to particular circumstances. Within the context of directive and non-directive roles, Batten (1967) suggested that there are a number of factors affecting this choice, including:

> what the worker sees as people's major needs, and his thoughts about people who have these needs; the way in which the worker sees himself: 'thus the more expert in diagnosing and meeting people's needs he feels himself to be, and the less he trusts the people he is working with to do this well enough for themselves, the more likely he is to choose a directive approach'; what the worker thinks will prove acceptable to the people he wants to work with.

Factors that affect role

In general, the choice of role might also be influenced by some or all of the following factors.

Type of work

Rothman (1974) has usefully suggested that his three models of community organisation (community work) practice are *primarily* associated with the following roles.

> *Locality development:*enabler, catalyst, coordinator, teacher of problem-solving skills and ethical values
> *Social planning:* fact-gatherer and analyst, programme implementer, facilitator
> *Social action:* activist, advocate, agitator, broker, partisan

Rothman is not suggesting that those roles are in practice or desirably confined to each mode of community work, or that the roles associated with, say, social planning are not appropriate or apparent in social action. Rather, he suggests that these roles are more salient than others in their respective modes of community work. It is clear that, in so far as any piece of work will incorporate aspects of each of the three models, then the worker will be called upon to play a large number of the salient roles.

Phases of work

We suggest that the phases or stages of neighbourhood work and point of development of the community group's activities are among the key determinants of the roles to be played by the neighbourhood worker. The degree of directiveness or activism of the worker should vary according to the early, middle and closing phases of a group's life. The same point can be made by looking at the worker's tasks in the different phases of intervention – it seems self-evident, for example, that the worker will need quite different roles in withdrawing from a group from those used in helping to recruit members to set it up.

The goals of the worker

The nature of the relationship between a worker's goals and the roles that she or he adopts is something that has received little attention in the community work literature. Rothman's discussion of the relationship between goals and roles provides one of the few analyses. He indicates that there is no *necessary* relationship between non-directiveness and process goals, on the one hand, and, on the other, between directiveness and product goals. He also argues that role directiveness is not undemocratic:

> It is not the *act* of giving goal direction that may be questionable, but rather the *way* it is given. Within this logic, the practitioner . . . may validly suggest, advocate, and stimulate, as long as the approach is a factual and rational one, conveyed without entering into personalities and invective, without expressing primarily personal motives and desires, without bringing overbearing pressure, and, most important of all, as long as the final decision is left with the citizen group in which ultimate authority resides – and this lay prerogative is manifestly conveyed.
>
> (Rothman, 1969)

The value of stressing the *way* of giving goal direction is to confirm the point that the worker must give advice and suggest direction in a way which does not impair the freedom of the group to decline that advice. How direction is given will vary according to the stage of development or sophistication of the group.

What the worker likes doing

We do not suggest that this is a major criterion to decide one's role predisposition because there are obvious risks to a group where a worker sticks stubbornly to roles that suit her likes and dislikes. We acknowledge one of the lessons from Alan Barr's research that 'Community workers cannot justify their interventions on the basis of their personal dispositions towards particular interests that have attracted their attention' (Barr, 1996: 163). Yet role effectiveness is in some way conditional upon the worker liking his or her role – and liking it from the point of view of its congruence with her values and feelings, as well as from satisfaction. What distinguishes the community worker is a disciplined use of self in her transactions with local groups – knowing when and how to contribute to the tasks and socio-emotional life of the neighbourhood group. This discipline may be contingent upon the worker being able, or having learnt, to *accept* the role and thus being able to function comfortably within it.

Agency constraints and opportunities

The neighbourhood worker's attempts to define roles must take into account, first, the expectations held of the role by her agency and colleagues, and, secondly, factors about an agency's values, structure and policies that the worker can anticipate influencing her role options. For example, a neighbourhood worker from a local authority department may not be able to adopt a high-profile or 'front-line' role in a group's negotiations with that authority. Equally as relevant as agency constraints are any expectations of a worker's role held within the local community – what local people think a worker should be doing and how she should carry out the work.

Role choice and role arenas

The notion of a continuum of directive/non-directive roles has been such a predominant influence in thinking about roles that it is very easy to fall into the trap of believing that a worker must be consistently directive or consistently non-directive. We suggest that the options about role that are open to the worker depend in large part on the nature of the *arena* in which she finds herself having to choose between roles. We suggest that there are three broad arenas, or situations, in which the worker will find herself and that each of these has its own opportunities for the choice of role by the worker. The three arenas are:

- relations with local people, either as individuals or in the group situation;
- dealings between the group and other organisations in its environment;
- transactions about the group within the worker's own agency, and between the worker and other agencies.

A worker can choose quite different roles according to the particular arena. It is possible for the worker to be a non-directive enabler in one situation, and a highly directive negotiator and advocate in another. We shall now explore these possibilities in more detail, though we are aware that these arenas are not so clear-cut and static in practice as we present them here.

Relations with local people

The directive/non-directive continuum seems appropriate only in considering role choice in relations with local people, and we suggest later that there are better ways of looking at role in respect of the two other arenas. Moreover, we believe that the degree of directiveness of the worker is a consideration that is largely relevant only to understanding *some* of the aspects of the worker's relations with local people, in particular the way in which the worker structures his or her contribution to group discussions and decision-making.

We see no value in being dogmatic or prescriptive about how directive or otherwise a worker should be. Her choice in this matter must above all else be guided by a sense of pragmatism, with the choice being heavily influenced by what the worker sees as the needs of the group or of the individual in the particular situation. There is probably a strong case for neighbourhood workers to be *predisposed* to non-directiveness, but this does not mean that the worker should reject more directive stances if these seem to be likely to be more helpful. The early stages of a group's life may call for a good deal of direct interventions by the worker, though in the last phase of a group the more appropriate stance might be that of non-directiveness.

Part of the difficulty that often faces students and workers about role choice is lack of clarity about what directiveness and non-directiveness mean. They suggest the basis of a continuum whose intermediate points remain unclear. In the next few pages, we propose to specify the different activities involved in directive and non-directive roles. First, let us start with directiveness, for degrees of directiveness have already been suggested by Rothman (1969).

DIRECTIVENESS

Rothman suggests three points on the directive side of the continuum. These are:

> *Channelling:* (strongly directive) 'The practitioner asserts a particular point of view with supporting arguments and documentation. He channels thinking directly toward a given goal.'
> *Funnelling:* (considerably directive) 'This practitioner gives a range of possible choices and subtly funnels thinking in a given direction by asserting his preference for a particular goal and the rationale for that choice.'
> *Scanning:* (mildly directive) 'This practitioner scans the range of possibilities related to solving a particular problem, presenting them impartially and on the basis of parity. He provides an orientation to goal selection, setting out the boundaries within which possible rational goal selection may take place.'

The need for workers to be strongly directive at times has increased in recent years. This is due principally, in our experience, to the need to respond to and challenge instances of discrimination – especially racial discrimination – manifested either within a community group or between a group and other community members. There are also situations where a worker is aware of a 'hidden agenda' of certain individuals and sees the need, in the interest of the group she or he is supporting, to challenge them. An example of this was observed by one of the authors in a meeting of local people and professionals in an area of Liverpool. The meeting had been called to plan a funding bid for a drugs prevention project. Three people in suits arrived at the meeting. The community worker knew that they belonged to the Church of Scientology and that they were preparing a separate bid to the same funding source. Firmly but calmly she insisted, with the support of other participants, that, because there was a conflict of interests, they leave the meeting. After some discussion, they agreed to this. Afterwards, people in the meeting commented on the skill of the worker and the correctness of the stance taken.

NON-DIRECTIVENESS

A great deal has been written about non-directiveness in community work and the classic texts are those of Batten (1967), the Biddle and Biddle (1965, 1967) and Ross (1967). For Batten, the essence of non-directiveness is

> to create sufficiently favourable conditions for successful group action without in any way infringing group autonomy either by making decisions for the group or by doing for its members anything that they could reasonably be expected to do, or learn to do, for themselves.

In general the worker does this by:

- trying to strengthen the incentives people have for acting together;
- providing information about how other groups have organised;
- helping people systematically to think through the problems they wish to deal with;
- suggesting sources of any needed material help and technical advice;
- helping to resolve any interpersonal difficulties between group members.

The Biddles develop their notion of non-directiveness by elaborating on the role of the community worker as *encourager*. It is extremely difficult to summarise the components of this role but it seems to comprise the activities of bringing people out of isolation, building optimism among local people, making internal conflict creative and 'making group life satisfying and productive', and helping people to use experts without surrendering their autonomy to them. The personal qualities that an encourager should seek to exemplify are also discussed by the Biddles.

Murray Ross describes three roles for the community worker – those of *guide, enabler* and *expert* – and sees them as highly compatible and mutually supporting. He provides a clear exposition of the desirable behaviours and attitudes associated with each of these roles. In particular, his account of the role of enabler is one of the fullest expositions of non-directiveness in neighbourhood work. The work of the enabler involves:

- focusing discontent on community conditions;
- encouraging organisation;
- nourishing good interpersonal relationships;
- emphasising common objectives.

We need to know, however, *how* the enabler carries out these aspects of his or her work, and Ross's comments on this are:

> As an enabler the worker seeks to facilitate the community process through listening and questioning; through identifying with, and in turn being the object of identification for, group leaders in the community; and by giving consistent encouragement and support to indigenous (people) striving with common problems. He does not lead; he facilitates local efforts. He does not provide answers; he has questions which stimulate insight. He does not carry the burden of responsibility for organisation and action in the community; he provides encouragement and support for those who do.
>
> (Ross, 1967)

Experience of practising neighbourhood work suggests that enabling is also about very practical forms of help to facilitate participation and collective action, such as providing information, transport, access to IT support, arranging meeting rooms and childcare.

The activity of *questioning* is central to the way in which the non-directive role is carried out, and to the way in which it is conceptualised by a number of the 'non-directive' writers. For Ross, questioning is a technique that the worker uses both to help the group in its 'here-and-now' discussions and 'to gain perspective, sense of movement, and fresh concern with long term objectives'.

Batten stresses that the purpose of questioning is to help the group to *think*, 'by structuring, enlarging, and systematising the thinking process of the group'. The worker might intervene in a discussion, says Batten, in order to:

- ensure that group members really are agreed about what they want to discuss;
- ensure that they consider a range of possibilities and not just one;
- keep discussion centred on one item at a time;
- ensure that discussion in the group is based on facts and not on assumptions about facts;
- ensure that the group is aware of factors it needs to take into account;
- help to assess the progress that has been made and what still remains to be done.

(Batten, 1967)

Questioning as a technique, however, is not confined to neighbourhood workers who work in a traditional non-directive way. It is an important element of dialogical education and the 'conscientisation' process associated with Paulo Freire. It is, too, a technique used by workers who have traditionally been seen as outside the non-directive camp. For example, Saul Alinsky (1971) stresses the value of 'guided questioning' to the organiser.

Having carried out this brief review of thinking on non-directiveness, we are now in a position to clarify further the role of the worker behaving in a non-directive fashion. Clearly it is possible to think of non-directiveness as a continuum ranging from, say, information collection to laissez-faire but we have chosen to emphasise types of interventions in group processes and discussions that exemplify the non-directive role of the neighbourhood worker. We suggest there are seven types of intervention to be associated with non-directiveness in the group situation:

Galvanising: The worker seeks to galvanise individuals or a group, stimulating their interest and their morale and mobilising them either to form a group or, if in one, to stick to working out its goals and tasks. The worker does this by the following means:

- *Supportive behaviour and interventions.* This involves interpersonal methods of working such as counselling, advising, building self-esteem and generally encouraging people to work through difficult situations;
- *Strengthening incentives for people to take action.* Batten suggests that the worker does this by helping people to restate their needs in terms of specific wants and goals to be achieved;
- *Inspiring people with a vision of what can be achieved in the neighbourhood by local people coming together.* Both Alinsky and Warren Haggstrom have written about the contribution of the worker's vision, and Haggstrom has written of its mobilising effects as follows:

An organiser must not only perceive how people are, but it is also essential that he be *unrealistic* in that he perceives people as they can be. Noting what is possible, the organiser projects this possibility and moves people to accept it and to seek to realise it. The organiser helps people to develop and live in an alternative reality in which their image of themselves and their abilities is enhanced . . . .. People are moved to accept the new world of which they catch a glimpse because it appears to be attainable in practice and intrinsically superior to the world in which they have been living.

(Haggstrom, 1970)

This way of describing the visionary qualities required by a neighbourhood worker may seem over-idealistic in the context of the most disadvantaged communities because often residents appear to have low expectations and an absence of a sense of rights. However, as Fiona Ballantyne argues, this kind of reality actually reinforces Haggstrom's point:

> In many ways neighbourhood workers need to hold on to their strong belief in the possibility of change and in the non-acceptance of the status quo. The importance of valuing people and seeing them as they could be brings neighbourhood workers into the world of possible dreams.

(Ballantyne, personal communication)

There is further discussion of galvanising in the next chapter.

Focusing: This activity by the neighbourhood worker helps to keep the group focused on the task at hand.

The focuser follows three rules:

- he does not get into competition with group members.
- he shows support (creates a positive environment) for any idea that a member voices (while trying to retain focus).
- he should keep interest at a high level, mainly through demanding and asking difficult questions.

Clarifying: The worker intervenes here in order to ensure that:

- people are clear about the purposes of the discussion, and the task the group is working on;
- the comments and questions of individual members are unambiguous and understood by all;
- real consensus has been reached before the group moves on to discuss another agenda item.

Summarising: The purpose of summarising is to help the group to take stock of discussions, and to assess how much progress has been made towards completing its task. The worker intervenes to condense the group's discussion to a few sentences. Summarising may be seen as an intervention that helps the movement of the group through the various stages of its discussion.

Gatekeeping: This type of intervention by the worker is designed to ensure that each of the members in the group has an opportunity to contribute to discussion. This means encouraging participants who say little and helping to limit the contributions of others who are more dominant in the discussion.

Mediating: This intervention seeks to resolve interpersonal disagreements between members that the worker believes are a threat to the group attaining its discussion objectives. Too much energy can be dissipated in a group on negative relationships between members.

Informing: The worker facilitates discussion in the group by acting as an informant about:

- resources and advice that the group might need to make decisions;
- facts that the group needs in its discussions;
- the experiences of other groups in reaching decisions about similar kinds of issues.

It must be emphasised that the aforementioned seven functions in the group process are not the prerogative of the neighbourhood worker or any other practitioner. They are functions that ought to be 'shared' among all the members of a group. We suggest only that it is through taking up one or several of these functions during a group meeting that the worker is able to contribute non-directively to the discussion. He is also modelling good discussion management behaviour which may be picked up by the group.

Dealings between the group and other organisations

The labels that conventionally define the role of the neighbourhood worker at the interface of the group and more formal and established organisations include broker, mediator, advocate, negotiator and bargainer. They immediately convey the sense of greater worker autonomy and activism, though it is not the case that the nature of these interface roles determines or predicts the roles the worker plays *within* the group situation. The worker may, of course, take or be given more of a leadership role at the interface but remain inside the boundary of non-directiveness in his or her relations with local people.

Neighbourhood groups have to deal with a number of other systems, including local authority departments, health agencies and voluntary organisations as well as other groups in the community. Such transactions might include meetings, deputations, petitions, demonstrations, holding a press conference, negotiating for money and other resources, and lobbying. For each of these transactions, the group and the worker must give thought to what role the worker will play. If there is to be a meeting with elected members about a particular issue, is the worker to come along? If so, will the worker play the role of observer/recorder, or will she be given the mandate to intervene as she thinks necessary?

The critical first step for group and worker to take in respect of the worker's role is to realise and accept that this question of role needs to be thought about, discussed and decided upon. It is all too easy in the rush and turmoil of preparing for a meeting to neglect to discuss the worker's contribution, if any (indeed, many groups are less than effective in such meetings largely because they have failed to discuss *member* roles adequately). It is especially important to be clear in what capacity the worker will be attending – as a representative of the group or of her agency?

The notion of representation is a helpful one in understanding the worker's role in dealings with other organisations. In most cases, the worker will be attending as a representative of the group, and indeed the members of a committee who go to a meeting are also representatives of that committee and of its wider constituency in the neighbourhood. Rice (1965) differentiated between three kinds of representation – observer, delegate and plenipotentiary – and these are helpful in understanding the neighbourhood worker's degree of activism and autonomy in negotiations between the group and other systems.

OBSERVER/RECORDER

Here the worker's job consists solely of observing and taking notes of what occurs. The neighbourhood group has not given her the mandate to express any views or intervene in the discussion. The worker's presence may also be a support to the group and an unsettling factor to 'the other side'.

DELEGATE

In this role, the worker is given a set piece to say, either at some agreed point in the transactions or at her discretion. For example, the worker might be asked by the group to present the statistical side of the case it is making to decision makers, and it is understood that the worker will confine her contribution to giving this information. The worker has no authority to go outside this brief.

PLENIPOTENTIARY

In this role, it is only the predetermined goals and policies of the group that provide limits on the negotiating power of the worker in transactions with other systems. The worker and perhaps the group members are given a flexible and open-ended mandate to contribute to the discussion as she thinks fit.

The final point to make about these three kinds of representation is that they can, of course, be used to understand the kind of mandate a committee or constituency will give to a delegation. Very often in neighbourhood work, delegations get into trouble with their committee, and the committee with its constituency, because the delegation was not given, and did not itself establish, whether it had observer, delegate or plenipotentiary powers in its negotiations with outside systems. The consequence of this absence of clarity is that delegations often commit their committees to courses of action when they were not empowered to do so.

Transactions about the group in the worker's agency

Neighbourhood workers are rightly wary of being put in the position of spokesperson or go-between for community groups. Yet in their own agency they may be asked to comment on some matter that concerns the community group they work with, or other agencies may contact them to give or to ask for information about the group. In most of these situations, the worker will attempt to get the inquirers to make direct contact with the local group, offering perhaps the mobile number or email address of the relevant officer. Within the group, the worker may be also seen as spokesperson or representative of her agency or even of the local authority, and again she may see her role as putting local people in direct contact with those agency staff who can best help them with the particular inquiry.

This re-routing function may constitute, together with the passing on of information and intelligence, the lowest level of activity for the worker in her agency setting. There is, however, a need to consider that opportunities for a more high profile role will often arise. For example, a practitioner working with homeless families may find herself in situations where she can promote their general and specific interests through contributions to agency discussions. The worker may be able to seize opportunities to promote an organisational or policy change that is in their interests, or a person working on play issues with a group may suddenly become aware of unallocated resources available in the department. In other words, situations will occur in which the neighbourhood worker will be pressured to make a decision that concerns the work of a group without being able fully to refer the matter back to the group. These may be the types of situation the worker would much prefer to avoid but there will be times when this is not possible. What is the worker to do? Make a bid to secure the unallocated resources for the group or sit quietly, because she has not been able to consult the group, and let the resources be put to some other use in the agency or community?

There is no easy answer or prescription for dealing with such situations but the fact that they occur ought to be discussed between the worker and the group. It might then be possible for each to establish guidelines to help the worker to handle better the linkage role between agency and group. The making explicit of the worker's status as an agency employee, and how she is to manage her roles of employee and community worker, serves another important purpose. It should help both the worker and the group not to be seduced into seeing the worker as just another group member, and to recognise the potential stress for the worker in feeling accountable both to her agency and to the community group. There is little value in the worker and the group 'pretending' that the worker is a full member because events will occur when the worker will have to say 'I'm sorry, but I can't do this with you', and this sudden revelation may undermine the confidence of the group.

There has been increasing evidence that experienced leaders of community groups have at times taken on the community worker role. This can be because they have seen, over the years, how different practitioners have worked and have become aware how they could carry out particular tasks. Or it can come about because of the need to fill a vacuum when a practitioner has left and has not been replaced. The phenomenon raises important questions concerning clarity of role and, in the context under discussion, the nature of representation at key meetings.

We have discussed three different arenas which suggest different role possibilities for the neighbourhood worker. The purpose has been to free our discussion (and the worker's choice of role) from the constraints that are imposed by both the traditional role labels and the blanket application of the directive/non-directive polarity. We now move to discuss the fourth element of working out what to do next.

Specifying the next moves

The neighbourhood worker must now use previously developed statements about problems, goals, skills and roles to decide how to move into, and carry out, the next task of making contact with local people in order to form a group or organisation around the salient issue or problem. In other words, the worker needs to think about and specify next steps as they seem predicted by earlier assessments and decisions.

Let us assume a worker has, when sorting out goals and priorities, decided to work with local people on the issue of play. She has given some preliminary thought to her own skills and experience in this task, and anticipated the variety of roles she may be called upon to take. The worker now has to decide and estimate *method*, *time* and *resources*. She has to ask herself: *how* will I organise local people and what time and resources will be demanded from me and other people? In addition, the worker might also anticipate any difficulties and resistances she might encounter, and how she will overcome or circumvent them. The planning tasks may be portrayed as follows:

Major objectives: To organise a group of local people around the issue of play.

Method: Here the worker must consider the alternatives open of identifying, meeting and encouraging people to form a group. The worker needs to evaluate the likely costs and benefits of each approach and technique, and specify what they will demand of her skills, time and other resources. Different methods of forming a group are discussed in the next two chapters.

Resistance: What factors can the worker anticipate will frustrate, hinder or delay intervention? There seem to be two categories: those within the community (e.g. apathy, suspicion and fragmentation) and those in her agency and other institutions (lack of mandate, support, understanding and facilities). Conversely, the worker should anticipate those factors that will help and facilitate intervention.

Circumvention: The worker then thinks about how to go round these resistances and remove the blockages. She may have to modify the original plan if she anticipates being able to do little about the predicted resistance.

Reporting and assessment: The worker must also plan how she will record her intervention to organise a group and the purposes for which she will record. One important purpose of record-keeping is to facilitate the monitoring and assessment of the intervention. The worker must be prepared to alter her problem choice, major objective and method if further contact with local people provides evidence to question her earlier assessments and decisions.

Summary

This chapter has stressed the importance of planning as an integral element of the neighbourhood work process. We are aware, however, of the possible dangers to action, in particular that preparation and planning can be used to put off and delay intervention. We have indicated already that the early stages are probably the most stressful for the neighbourhood worker and some workers may be tempted to prolong planning in order to postpone engagement with action. Clearly, workers and agency supervisors need to be alert to this possibility.

On the other hand, we suggest that planning and reflection of the kind we have described in this chapter may be a way of mitigating the stress of the first stages of neighbourhood work by guiding the worker through the various activities and stages of her intervention. However, no amount of planning and preparation will enable the worker to predict all the variables in a turbulent community environment that will shape and distort her work, and so the worker's guided intervention needs to remain responsive to the influences and events encountered when making contact with local residents.

References

Alinsky, S. (1971) *Rules for radicals*, New York: Random House.
Barr, A. (1996) *Practising community development. Experience in Strathclyde*, London: CDF Publications.

Batten, T. R. (1967) *The non-directive approach in group and community work*, Oxford: OUP.

Biddle, W. W. and Biddle, L. J. (1965, 1967) *Encouraging community development*, New York: Holt, Rinehart & Winston.

Haggstrom, W. C. (1970) 'The psychological implications of the community development process', in L. J. Cary (ed.) *Community development as a process*, Columbia: University of Missouri Press.

Rice, A. K. (1965) *Learning for leadership*, London: Tavistock.

Ross, M. (1967) *Community organisation* (2nd edn), London: Harper & Row.

Rothman, J. (1969) 'An analysis of goals and roles in community organisation practice', in R. Kramer and H. Specht (eds) *Readings in community organisation practice* (1st edn), Englewood Cliffs, NJ: Prentice-Hall.

Rothman, J. (1974) 'Three models of community organisation practice', in F. M. Cox *et al.* (eds) *Strategies of community organisation* (2nd edn), Itasca, IL: Peacock.

6   Making contacts and bringing people together

Making contact: but for what reasons?	Ways of making contact
The process of making contact	Contacts initiated by the worker
Preparing for the contact	Contacts initiated by residents
The contact	Conclusions
After the contact	

This chapter is about the neighbourhood worker making contact with local people. The task of the worker is to meet residents in order to identify their interest in collective action and the possible contributions they might make, and to bring them together with other individuals. The purpose is to help people form a group. Chapter 7 deals with the transformation of a group into an organisation that represents a constituency on whose behalf the organisation will act.

Methods and skills in making contact with people are essential through the whole neighbourhood work process, so we must stress that *many of the ideas and techniques discussed as part of this phase are relevant within all the other phases of the process.* The particular phase of making contacts in order to get people into a group is, however, especially crucial for the worker. Failure here means that the process of getting people organised can hardly start. The ways in which the worker initially relates to residents and helps them explore the possibilities of collective action are likely to affect their later development and goals as a community organisation.

Encouraging people to form a group or network demands a variety of skills on the part of the worker. It is, too, a phase of neighbourhood work in which the worker will again feel isolated and vulnerable, moving between states of elation and depression as residents respond positively or negatively to her encouragement. The worker is at risk of assimilating the doubts and despair that are voiced by both local people and agency staff, and she will often be harassed by an internal need and an external expectation (again from local residents and agency workers) to achieve something.

There are other sources of stress in this phase of the work. The worker may have strong doubts about her legitimacy and credibility for intervening in a community. She may also feel uncertain about the best ways of making contact with people. She wants answers to the following sorts of questions: How do I approach people? Do I knock on a door or stop someone in the street? How will I introduce myself? Will they understand what I say? Will they talk to me? What business do I have to confront local people about issues in their area? A female worker may feel that while it may

DOI: 10.4324/9781003310006-6

be alright for male workers to knock on doors and approach strangers, what do they think when they see me, a woman, engaged in these activities? The neighbourhood can so easily become for the worker an undifferentiated and unreceptive entity, some of whose members may be openly hostile and rejecting of the worker's efforts to make contacts.

Many of these doubts and anxieties are stimulated by the fact that most workers *are* outsiders and strangers. It may be that neighbourhood workers do not always appreciate the extent to which they are strangers to the community they wish to serve. Many workers may have a strong sense of identification with the needs and problems of the inhabitants of an area but may be unaware that their feelings of attachment are not reciprocated; workers may not realise that their identification and commitment do little to mediate between their status as an outsider and the continuing problems (and distrust of professionals) of the neighbourhood.

It is natural for workers to assume that there is in the community an understanding and appreciation of their work that will easily overcome suspicion about their motivation to help. The very closeness of relationships that often develops between a worker and a neighbourhood group can lead even the most experienced worker to fudge the marginality of her position with local people, which exists even when she is well known to the members of a group, and even after she has been tested and 'accepted'. How much more marginal is the position of the worker at the time she attempts to initiate contact with local residents!

Apprehension – even fear – of what will be encountered will clearly vary with the type of person the worker is, and the kind of neighbourhood in which he or she seeks to intervene. But being scared to one degree or another may be an inevitable part of this phase of the work:

> The extent to which it happens depends on whether the worker is relatively new to the area or not, whether she is a woman working with young men, whether she is a black or Asian worker operating in a predominantly white neighbourhood or vice versa. . . . The lone worker always needs to take safety measures such as a mobile phone, personal alarm and informing someone where you are and when you expect to be back.
>
> (Smalle, personal communication)

Part of the apprehension has to do with uncertainty as to who to make contact with and an awareness of the range of possibilities. This applies especially in multicultural communities:

> Working with diversity in a multicultural/multi-faith setting requires the worker to try to understand and work with a range of practices. This does not mean, necessarily, that she accepts and agrees with all practices. It is an acknowledgement of the right of others to hold, for example, certain religious views. Workers may be called to cover their heads, take off their shoes, sit on the floor or not expect eye contact with someone of the opposite sex. These are all concessions which show some acceptance of working in a diverse neighbourhood. Investing a little time in preparing for making contact in a multicultural/multi-faith setting is time well spent.
>
> (Smalle, personal communication)

A worker's apprehension when making contact in the community can easily cut across the need to keep the possibilities of participation very open:

> These fears work on most organisers to make them very susceptible to thinking the people they meet in the community who are sympathetic are the people to listen to and work with. I can't count the number of times I have wandered into communities to find the people who were supposed to be building a mass organization mucking around with pious, middle-class clergymen or teenagers.
>
> (Von Hoffman, 1972)

Von Hoffman's comment is suggestive of yet another source of doubt and anxiety for the worker in this stage of the process. The task of identifying leaders or, more generally, of recruiting people to form a group may appear to the worker to depend too much on chance and opportunism rather than on judgement and skills. Success in making the right contacts may seem determined by many factors outside a worker's control. A worker who happens to be in the right pub at the right time on the right day may meet the indigenous community leader most able to take forward the organisation of a group; if the worker is not there, the group may go forward in a completely different way, with different personalities and interests.

But how does the worker *know* when she or he meets the people most likely to help to get a group going? What criteria does the worker use to assess people's likely contribution to collective action? And is it the worker's business, anyway, to select out people – is neighbourhood work not supposed to be about enabling the least motivated and able to take part in community affairs? Von Hoffman again indicates some of the difficulties for the worker:

> Plucking out 'natural leaders' by dint of casual observation and conversation is very chancy. I recall having picked a number of these on-first-sight gems and I also recall spending months kicking myself for having done so . . . The leaders in the third month of an organisation's life are seldom the leaders in the third year; a few leaders, ourselves included, are really all-purpose; and the best organisations create a 'collective leadership'. The first leadership is usually the closest leadership at hand. It is usually selected in the enthusiasm of the first campaign, because it is available. You don't have a choice and you have to go with what you've got. But you will notice too that the reasons for your picking the first leaders (and you know it's you who picks them) say nothing about how they will wear out over a period of time. The lesson I draw from this is that at the beginning keep the organisation very loose, and spread the responsibilities and the conspicuous places around. This permits you, and the new membership that you are supposed to be recruiting, to judge the talent, and it keeps things sufficiently porous so that new talent isn't blocked off. Nothing is more absurd than an organization that's six months old, without a dime in the treasury and a membership that can fit in a Volkswagen, having a cemented-in, piggy leadership. Vested interests are only tolerable when they are protecting something of value, not fancy organisational charts, letterheads, and research programmes. Don't laugh. This kind of thing is a clear and present danger.
>
> (Von Hoffman, 1972)

We continue the discussion about the identification of leadership in the next chapter. The need to identify and commit oneself to people is not the only source of concern for the worker who has, too, to help residents to identify an interest in a problem or issue. The worker will wonder what criteria to use to decide on what is a 'good' problem or issue to work with.

How the worker makes judgements about people and issues highlights a major 'policy' decision that workers will often face in these opening moves of neighbourhood work. There seem to be two different situations that may confront a worker as the process of group formation begins.

The first is where the worker's goal is to enable a specific group of people to organise for community action – the worker has a sense of whom to organise (e.g. residents of a housing estate) and the tasks are to determine the pragmatic means by which to do so, including the identification of the issues around which people are likely to organise.

In the second situation the worker's goal is to generate some group action in respect of a specific need – the worker wants to do something about a particular problem or issue around which people can mobilise (e.g. poor housing, lack of recreational facilities). The major tasks are the identification and recruitment of appropriate individuals, groups and organisations. In both situations, the worker has to build up contacts with local residents, not just as individuals, but also perhaps as members of neighbourhood groups that are already in existence.

The issue of whether to work through an existing organisation or to by-pass it and help create another is often a testing one for the neighbourhood worker. The issue is crucial in a 'closed' community like a housing estate where there would seem to be little 'room' for a new organisation, and where the attempt to generate something new may lead to animosities not only between the worker and the existing group but also between neighbours and friends.

On the other hand, a new group may be preferable if existing groups are unrepresentative of the goals and ambitions of the community, or where it pursues interests that do not address the concerns of most people. A typical example is a tenants' association that refuses to enlarge on its role of running a bar and other social facilities and will not take up housing and other issues of concern to the tenants. Some existing groups may also be prejudiced against the interests of minority sections of the community, and these can be protected only by forming alternative organisations. The difficulty for the neighbourhood worker is that he or she may be acutely aware of the deficiencies of existing groups, but be just as aware of the pitfalls in trying to circumvent them. It will be important to set out the positives and negatives of each option, relating them to relevant values and purposes.

Making contact: but for what reasons?

We are concerned primarily in this chapter with making contact on a person-by-person basis. We see other forms of contact-making, such as by letter, mobile phone or email, as being more relevant when they precede and thus facilitate personal contact and understanding. What we have to consider is how the worker sets about *engaging* with potential members of a community group, or with actual members of an existing group(s).

At one level it seems self-evident why the neighbourhood worker has to make contact with local people: he cannot carry out his work if he does not make relationships with them. But there are more specific purposes behind this phase of making contact.

Giving people the opportunity to get to know the worker and to form some initial assessment of the worker as a person. This is especially important in isolated communities in which local people may be reluctant to engage with 'incomers'. This was the case for Jo Laverick, a community worker with the Community Council of Northumberland in the coastal area of the county. Her previous community work experience had been in inner-city areas and she was aware of the contrast with the rural area where there was a resistance to change:

> She adopted a 'softly-softly' approach, politely introducing herself to parish councillors and waiting for an invitation. A few asked her to speak at one of their meetings and, gradually, the phone started ringing with people requesting advice and information. Jo made herself very accessible and made it clear that she was there to work in the area on local people's behalf. By promoting herself as a service, she found she could help them to work out how best to use her time. These negotiations with groups formed a valuable part of the community development process. Jo was able to develop rapport and build trust so that she and the groups created a working relationship.
>
> (Wilson and Wilde, 2001: 24)

Local people need to find out how reliable the worker is or is likely to be, where his loyalties lie, how he sees the neighbourhood and understands the people who live in it and the problems they face, and how he responds to different kinds of people and situations in the neighbourhood. They also need to learn about various aspects of the worker's personality, beliefs and values that are important to local people or provide clues as to how useful the worker is going to be to any group that might form.

Presenting information about the worker's role, organisation and what he or she has to offer. Among the factors that some people will take into account when weighing up the costs and benefits of getting involved in community action will be their understanding of the part and role the worker will play. They may also be interested in the resources that can be opened up through the worker's own role and skills, and of any resources he or she may be able to bring. The worker must be specific and frank enough for people to be able to assess his potential contribution; yet not so intrusive that it seems to be more salient than the roles, skills and resources of the community, and not so dominating that it fosters a sense of dependence.

The difficulties facing a worker attached to a neighbourhood work project are that people may find it hard to understand the origins and function of the project, whereas for workers employed, for example, in a high-profile regeneration programme, the problem is almost a contrary one: people will often have quite well-formed views on the function of the programme. The worker may have difficulty in describing his role in ways that distinguish his particular contribution from those of other staff from the programme already known to residents. He may also become the focus of anger and enquiry, possibly placing him in a difficult position.

The effective presentation by the worker of self, role and organisation (as well, perhaps, as his previous experience) will contribute to establishing his identity – 'getting a licence to operate'. The concreteness and credibility of his identity will depend on conclusions about him that people derive both from the information presented about his person, role and sponsor, and also on the *way* it is presented. Not only will people take clues about him from such things as dress, language and lifestyle but the answers that the worker gives to people's questions such as 'What's in it for him?', 'What's he really after?', 'Who is paying him to do this and why?' must be acceptable within the experience of the community.

Motivating, or galvanising, residents to consider the possibilities of community action Galvanisation comprises a number of activities including developing people's awareness about issues in an area, exploring the costs and benefits of collective action, alerting people to the range of skills and resources they have or that are available to them, and motivating them by establishing a sense of their general competence and confidence. It is not enough for people to become persuaded only of the worker's skills and competence.

Galvanisation involves both reflection and vision. Reflection, meaning an internal process of conceptualisation and reasoning, is a means through which people and groups overcome what Rowbotham (1974) has called a 'paralysis of consciousness' and become able to understand, conceptualise and articulate what goes on around them and impinges on their social, economic and political lives. Reflection of this kind may produce an understanding of how to intervene to affect these forces, and to predict, control and overcome them.

Techniques to facilitate reflection have been developed and used by community workers. Alinsky (1971), in particular, is well known for his repertoire of interventions designed to stimulate people into a thinking awareness of their situation. Much of his writing emphasises the importance of reflection and he argues, for instance, that

> the function of the organiser is to raise questions that agitate, that break through the accepted pattern ... [to raise] ... the internal questions within individuals that are so essential for the revolution which is external to the individual.

Citizens UK (part of the community organising movement) has taken forward Alinsky's ideas within the United Kingdom. It starts with the recognition that change can only come about when communities come together to compel public authorities and businesses to respond to the needs of ordinary people. It supports communities to build power by identifying and training leaders, bringing them together and organising campaigns. Learning and reflection are central to the approach taken by Citizens UK.

Reflection enables people to understand the situations that limit them and to attempt to overcome them. Vision follows on from reflection – increased consciousness of me-in-this-situation can lead to a vision of me-in-another-situation in the future.

Effective action is contingent upon local people being able to conceive of themselves as 'new' people – a conception of themselves working at tasks, taking on roles and exercising skills and knowledge in ways previously unimaginable to them. The neighbourhood worker's task is to help people to articulate a desired future state of affairs (such as better housing, a less polluted environment) and then to work with them to realise it. The challenge facing the worker, however, is that before people become organised, group members are often not visionary. They may perceive something is wrong, but often they do not know what they want to do by way of improving the situation, or how to go about it. The worker's task, then, is to develop in people a capacity for visionary thought, to help them cross what Freire has called 'the frontier which separates being from being more'.

The neighbourhood worker will often be purposively catalytic in galvanising group members to cross the frontier between 'being and being more'. There is a long and rich tradition of neighbourhood workers playing this role. The sociologist Richard Sennett goes back to the contribution made by Jane Addams at the Hull House settlement in Chicago at the beginning of the twentieth century. The organisers anticipated the approach taken later by Alinsky and others, focusing on the everyday experience of people, sharing the associational informality, providing simple ground rules but also challenging people to become involved in the future of their neighbourhood: 'The community organizer had, and has, to engage poor people who feel paralysed, whether as foreigners or simply losers in the capitalist game' (Sennett, 2012: 53). The worker can galvanise people by using her or his own vision of a better world to inspire them.

Moving people to accept a 'new world' requires at least three things of the neighbourhood worker. First, that he works with residents to develop appropriate organisation and decision-making processes; second, that he works with them to transform visionary statements into operational goals; and third, that he helps people to see leadership as located not just in himself but also in themselves and other members of the group. The skills that are required of the neighbourhood worker are not just those of knowing when and how to inspire people by sharing his vision and enthusiasm about their capabilities; but also those of doing so without appearing unrealistic or naive, and without seeming to impose his preconceptions about what the specific goals and strategies of the community effort might be.

Finally, increasing the worker's knowledge of people and their lives in the neighbourhood. This has two essential aspects. First, that of consolidating information about residents that was gathered in the earlier data-gathering phase of the intervention. Second, encouraging people to form a group around the issue or grievance in question; and, in particular, looking for residents who might occupy key leadership positions in any group that is formed.

In summary, we suggest that the important purposes to be achieved in the phase of making contact are to give and receive information about oneself and residents; to establish one's identity and identification with local people; to create rapport and the basis of trust and understanding; to affect attitudes and motivations about individuals' competence and the potential of collective action; to identify points of contact and intervention of mutual interest, and thus to clarify areas of 'goal convergence' between oneself and residents; and to begin to describe a provisional agenda for the involvement of worker and residents in the formation of a group. All of these indicate the substantive difference between making contact at this stage in the neighbourhood work process and the more limited engagement with the community described in Chapter 3.

The process of making contact

It should be evident by now that making contact is about verbal and non-verbal communication – it is a process of discussion, dialogue, questioning, listening and understanding. Contacts with local people may be differently perceived as 'conversations' or 'interviews'. If a worker sees them as conversations, they may be viewed more as a pleasurable activity, an art form, in which the social and work aspects of the contact are hard to separate out. The tendency to view contacts as conversations rather than interviews will be strengthened by feelings that the notion of an 'interview' jars with the worker's perception of the participatory, even peer, basis of contacts with local people.

Seeing contacts as interviews alerts one to the need to plan and prepare for them, to see them primarily as an instrumental and not a social activity, and to associate them with specific techniques and skills for carrying them out effectively. This approach to contacts is put most strongly by Brager and Specht. Referring their readers to the 'considerable material on the uses and techniques of interviewing in the literature', they write:

> interviewing may be distinguished from conversation on three important grounds: (1) it is *goal-oriented*, that is, the worker has a purpose, something that he wishes to come out of the contact; (2) it is *self-conscious* in that he is thoughtful about the interaction and his own role in it; and (3) it is *focused*, that is, the worker selects his questions and responses in the context of his purposes. Although the above may sound imposing and overformal, experienced interviewers can be friendly and warm, if required, without violating these strictures.
>
> (Brager and Specht, 1973)

The polarisation of views about whether contacts are conversations or interviews is helpful only if it enables us to recognise that contacts should be seen as embodying elements of both conversation and interview. Contact-making in neighbourhood work ought to be friendly, sociable, caring and receptive, as well as focused, purposeful and goal-directed. A balance has to be achieved between these elements. There is no point in the worker who is looking for information so structuring the contact that the other person becomes hostile and the worker fails to establish rapport and the basis for continuing work. On the other hand, there is limited value in a contact where the worker and other person get on famously together but the worker fails to acquire the information that he or she wants.

We suggest that the process of contact-making may helpfully be seen as comprising three stages.

Preparing for the contact

This consists of the following planning or preparation activities.

Selecting people to talk to, and the sequence in which to do so
Time can be wasted in talking with the 'wrong' people (wrong, perhaps, because with a bit of foresight you might have seen they could not add to what other people have already told you). Goodwill can be endangered by omitting to see people who think you *ought* to see them; and feathers and thus cooperativeness can be ruffled if there's a pecking order in the neighbourhood and you contacted people 'out of order'.

Selecting a setting in which to meet people
Two considerations should guide the selection of the setting. First, the purpose of the meeting. If the worker wants an extended and perhaps confidential

discussion, a noisy crowded pub with its distractions for the other person of friends and neighbours may not be the best place. Such a setting would be appropriate, however, if the worker wanted to use the meeting to get to know other people. Second, local attitudes to meeting places should be followed: a particular pub or café may not be a 'respectable' place to meet, or residents may feel reluctant to invite a relative stranger into their homes, or it may be assumed by some people that it is only acceptable to meet in a public building such as a community centre.

Deciding what you want to get out of the contact.

Is it information about some community issue or event, or the presentation of oneself as an interested and resourceful worker, or change in the other person's attitudes and behaviour, or introductions to other people in the area? Of course, the worker may have a number of goals for the contact, and so will have to decide which of them has priority.

Deciding on the means through which you will achieve the goals of the meeting.

Are there points of influence you can bring to bear to get the information or interest that you seek? What questions do you have to ask to get the information you seek from the other person? What will you be prepared to give to the other person in return for the help he or she can give?

Deciding on how you will present yourself, your agency and your interests.

This involves trying to anticipate, and thus minimise, any negative forces that may be at work in the meeting that derive from factors such as the personal attributes of the worker (e.g. age, sex, race), the status of the agency, and the other person's previous experience of neighbourhood work. The worker must also anticipate and make the most of positive forces in the situation. In brief, the worker must think how to manage her image in contact with different local people, though this does not entail giving up her integrity or behaving unlike her real self. Von Hoffman provides some interesting comments on image management and the way in which the organiser comes across to local people:

People may admire youth, they may praise, they may believe that youth is showing the way in which age should follow, but they are very, very reluctant to trust youth with anything of immediate value. Impressions do count.

'I'll mention clothes. It is one thing to wear overalls in Mississippi where many of the people actually do wear them – it is another to wear them as an occasional stunt in a big Northern city. To indulge in peculiarities of dress and speech simply makes you look like faddists'.

Drop as much of your excess ideological baggage as you can . . . don't act like cultists. If you are a vegetarian, keep it to yourself, hide it, because there are a certain number of butchers in the community, and you want them in the organisation too.

(Von Hoffman, 1972)

A further aspect of anticipating the contact is that of rehearsing it, though without detracting from the spontaneity that must be present. Contact may be rehearsed through discussing it with a colleague or through role play.

The contact

The task of the neighbourhood worker in any contact with local people is both to establish rapport and to achieve the outcomes for the contact that he has previously specified. Establishing rapport may itself be the goal, and it is doubtful that other goals (such as getting information about a community issue) would be achieved without some rapport between the worker and the other person. Brager and Specht have defined some of the elements of establishing rapport in a community work setting. These elements are that the worker is able to be accepting of others, to empathise, to tolerate feedback (about, for instance, himself, his intentions or his agency), to accept views that are unacceptable socially or to the worker, and to be able to 'speak the language' of the people though aware of the dangers of being patronising and ingratiating (Alinsky's phrase of 'speaking within the experience of the community' is a better one).

It may be difficult to think about rapport in a purposeful way. To do so seems to conflict with views that rapport is essentially to do with the 'chemistry' between two people, something that is outside the influence of the people concerned. It may seem inappropriate to think that there may be things one can do – guidelines to follow – that maximise positive and minimise negative rapport. Thinking in these terms might also be distasteful to workers who detect undertones of manipulation. For these and other reasons more may be learnt about establishing rapport from the field of participant observation.

Bearing in mind the twin tasks of establishing rapport and conducting the contact in such a way that the worker achieves the outcomes he or she has specified, we suggest that the actual contact with the other person may be seen as comprising the following activities.

Crossing the boundary

This may be that of a person's flat, or the entrance to the local temple. Different kinds of boundary pose different kinds of problems and challenges to different workers. The main task in boundary crossing is to take stock of the immediate environment in which the contact is to happen. The worker must decide on how to cope with factors in the environment that, for instance, may detract from the value of the contact. For example, in someone's home, there may be a noisy television in the room or a group of children at play, both of which might distract the attention of the worker and other person; the seating arrangements may be inappropriate; or there may be friends and neighbours present and the worker may not be sure how they will affect the progress of the contact.

Introducing oneself

Neighbourhood workers may be uncertain about how detailed, frank and specific their introductions should be. Some will see an emphasis on introductions as working against establishing rapport and a sense of ease, while others would feel that introductions are important so that the other person is aware of the nature and implications of the contact. The worker must introduce himself and his agency and give the other person an idea of what his purposes are, and why the other person has been chosen to be interviewed. It might help, too, to suggest the possible areas for discussion in the interview. Our experience from our skills workshops was that workers tended to give either too little information or too much. In giving too much information too soon the worker risks swamping the other person with data that are not heard or understood and will thus serve to confuse rather than inform.

Setting the contract for the contact

In many meetings with local people both they and the worker may want to discuss the terms on which the contact is taking place. The other person may want to know what use the worker is going to make of the outcomes of the contact (e.g. with whom is the information to be shared?) and be able to raise issues of confidentiality. The other person may wish to explore what they are 'being committed to' simply through the act of having a meeting with the worker. The worker may want to make it clear that he is not being committed to any course of action by virtue of talking with the other person about community issues.

Seeing the contact through

This refers to the main body of the discussion in which the worker seeks to achieve the goals that have been set for the contact. The worker asks questions, probes, stimulates reflection and discussion, throws in ideas and suggestions, establishes understanding with the other person, and integrates verbal communication with appropriate behavioural responses and cues. But the worker also listens and attends to what the other person is saying, trying to remember what he is being told, and negotiating and clarifying the meaning of what is said. He also pays attention to non-verbal communication.

The problem of remembering what has occurred in a contact is often a pressing one for workers in situations where it is not desirable or feasible to take notes or record on tape. In most cases, note-taking is acceptable; indeed it suggests that what is being said is taken seriously and validated. It is best, however, to ask permission. Comprehensiveness and accuracy of what is remembered can be developed through training and experience. We suggest the following devices to help recall conversations:

- Look for 'key words' in your subject's remarks.
- Concentrate on the first and last remarks in each conversation.
- Leave the setting as soon as you have observed as much as you can accurately remember.
- Make notes as soon after the contact as possible, perhaps using a laptop or electronic notepad.
- Do not talk with anybody about the contact until you have made notes.
- Make your notes up after each contact, and do not wait until the end of the day to write up a number of contacts.

Recall can also be facilitated by trying, towards the end of the contact, to summarise and clarify with the other person the major points that emerged in the discussion. This is also a way of reducing the risk of misrepresenting what has been said and agreed to between the worker and the other person.

It is also useful towards the end of the contact for the worker to focus more on consolidating his rapport with the other person than on pursuing the information he wants. This emphasis on rapport should help in providing the basis for further and continuing contacts with the other person.

After the contact

The activities of the worker after the end of the contact seem to comprise the following:

- *Recalling and writing up the contact* – noting what has been obtained, areas discussed and points of agreement and disagreement. The worker might also record any further action that may need to be taken as a result of the contact.
- *Informing others of the contact or passing on ideas and information that is generated (where appropriate).*
- *Following up the contact* – by sending (where appropriate) 'back-up' information about the worker and his interests; and encouraging the other person in any tasks he or she has agreed to do as a result of the contact.

We have referred already to the importance of taking note of the environment or setting in which contact-making is carried out. We want, too, to draw attention to other kinds of factors of which the worker ought to take account. Factors like the time of the day and the weather, for example, will affect the success of contacts that a worker makes with people on a street or on their doorsteps. The 'culture' of an area, and particularly its attitudes to strangers and outsiders, will bear on a worker's attempts to make contact with local people. We identified earlier the degree of 'closeness' and isolation of communities that affect the interventions of workers.

The physical design of 'closed' and 'open' housing areas will determine the type and quality of the worker's attempts to meet people and bring them together. We hope the reader will also consider how attempts at organising people are similarly influenced by other kinds of physical environments, particularly the layout and design of houses in estates, and the way factors like the horizontal or vertical patterning of roads, and the siting of amenities, may affect interchange between houses, streets and parts of a community.

Ways of making contact

It now seems appropriate to consider some of the different ways of initiating contacts with local people that are available to neighbourhood workers. The examples we give ought to be seen as illustrations, for we do not suggest that what we describe is comprehensive or that any of the techniques portrayed are necessarily right for all the situations in which workers find themselves. We would like our presentation of the different ways of making contact to be viewed in two lights: first, as an initial attempt to compile an inventory or repertoire of methods available, from which the worker must choose for the purposes in hand; and, second, as an indication that most of the methods we describe are important areas in which practitioners should have some skill and confidence.

An important feature of the way neighbourhood workers initiate relationships with local people is that they will often 'reach out' to where people are, taking the initiative and the first steps in making the contact. There are a number of reasons for this, including the fact that neighbourhood workers do not ordinarily operate on the basis of referrals, and some communities may not be 'aware' of needs and the possibilities open to them through collective action. Often people will need help to understand and challenge the problems and forces that affect their lives. Even if individuals are aware of their needs, they may not perceive them as being the same as, or relating to, the problems of other individuals in the community.

There seem to be two aspects in the process of making local contacts, and it is a matter for the worker to judge whether they occur simultaneously or sequentially. In the first, the worker knows in advance who it is she wishes to see. The worker has a list of local people whom she sets out to meet. There are a number of ways in which this list will be compiled: the worker will have on it the names of officers of existing groups in the community, those who were interviewed whilst collecting data and expressed interest in the work or some issue or community problem, those mentioned by local people whom the worker 'ought' to see, and, finally, residents whose interest in a particular aspect of community affairs has been mentioned in local newspapers and on deputations to the council. The worker may also have the names and addresses of people given by colleagues.

The second aspect of making contacts has to do with local people who are not 'known' or already affiliated to some grouping or organisation. In a sense, the worker wishes to reach out to, or to be reached by, the 'ordinary person in the street'. Depending on approach, the worker's method of contacting these people (i.e. the bulk of the population) will be haphazard and random and the people she will come into contact with will not be predictable. It is this second aspect of making contacts that we wish especially to examine further.

In order to do this, it is helpful to conceive of a continuum formed by the question: who initiates the contact? At one end of the continuum we identify contacts initiated by the worker; at the other end, contacts initiated by residents. The distinction between worker and resident-initiated contacts must be regarded as an aid to learning and as an attempt to impose some conceptual order on the array of opportunities open to the worker.

Contacts initiated by the worker

There are a variety of ways in which the worker can take the initiative and we describe some of these here.

Street work

Here the street (or courtyard outside a block of flats) is the setting for the contact. The worker who is 'street working' has much in common with the approach of detached youth workers and will often share a similar uncertainty:

> I tried to cover the patch at all different times of the day and night, so that I could soak up the flavour, and see if particular patterns emerged about where young people went at certain times or on certain days. This meant that, on many occasions, I did not meet anyone to talk to, and it was in these moments I wondered about what I was doing and if there was any purpose to my wanderings.
>
> (Wild, 1982: 23)

As Mark Smith, commenting on this passage, points out, it is crucial to go beyond simply observing the neighbourhood and its residents:

> It is through continuing conversations with people that workers can both enhance their local knowledge and engage in the central elements of their task. They are there not simply to learn about the area but to intervene.
>
> (Smith, 1994: 15)

Street work may be done at its best when the weather is kind; streets may often not contain a cross-section of a community's population but only a part of it; the variety and quality of contacts will depend upon what kind of environment the street is part of (street work in the villages and small towns of the South Wales valleys, for instance, will be different from that among densely populated tower blocks in east London).

The purpose of street work is to gain information and get people interested in organising. One approach to this task is that of 'snow-balling' – the process of working with individuals who build up a nucleus of friends and neighbours around a particular interest. From there, chains of contact can build up a wider constituency.

An altogether different style is to work with people in aggregate on the street which becomes, in effect, the setting for meetings, discussion groups, theatre and other events that stimulate discussion and an interest in organising. A play worker involved in consulting adults and children about traffic-calming techniques made use of Planning for Real principles to involve them – Planning for Real is a participatory planning technique (www.planningforreal.org.uk).

With other staff, the play worker arranged for models to be placed in certain streets so that children and adults could visualise possibilities and develop ideas from initial reactions contained in the results of a questionnaire. The results in terms of interest and participation were positive.

This example is helpful because it suggests a *planned and structured* approach to street work, particularly through the use of leaflets and the prior discussion of the strategy with residents. Attendance at the street meeting made fewer demands on participants than turning out to a 'traditional' public meeting, it involved children of all ages as well as adults, it capitalised on people's affiliation to their street, and it benefited from the visibility of the event, that is, the meeting was an inclusive activity and residents may have been encouraged to attend by seeing that their neighbours were present.

Jane Jacobs' book *The Death and Life of Great American Cities* (Jacobs, 1972) has been a classic text for planners and architects, many of whom are committed to neighbourhood planning and to using participatory methods. However, it is her insights on the function of the street in promoting and controlling social interaction between residents, and between them and strangers, that have been shown to be a useful antidote to fears that the urban street is necessarily a hard, merciless place of confrontation and rejection.

Yet there are problems for the practitioner in street working. On the street his or her role is ambiguous and people do appear to be rushing along pavements with great purpose, defying the worker to interrupt their pace and their thoughts. Some people, too, will outrightly reject an approach from a stranger, while others are suspicious and defensive about talking to someone they do not know. On the other hand, it is mostly the case that people are more friendly, interested and cooperative than they look! And there are ways in which the worker can help to reduce people's defensiveness such as, for example, standing at a bus stop or carrying a street map and looking uncertain about directions and places. Inevitably, the growth of 'chugging' and Big Issue vendors gives a different feel to street work.

There are three other aspects of street work that we have not mentioned yet. First, there is the use of pubs, cafés, shops and so on, in which to meet people. Second, there is making contact with people at points where the worker knows they are to be found, for example, older people in luncheon clubs, and claimants in and outside the local Jobcentre Plus offices. Third, there is door-to-door knocking, in which the worker arrives 'cold' on the doorstep or has leafleted the houses in advance to say that she will be calling. The leaflet might say something about the worker, her agency and her interests in talking with local people. The information the worker puts on a leaflet about herself, and whether a leaflet is used at all, will depend on her assessment of whether it will be helpful given what the worker knows about the neighbourhood.

Making contacts through knocking at doors may also be facilitated by an indirect approach. That is, the worker knocks on a door in order to distribute a leaflet or a community newspaper, waiting for views on the area to develop from more general discussion of the leaflet or newspaper. Indeed, the newspaper itself may be used to generate discussion if the worker draws attention to its contents. Finally, the worker who wishes to knock on doors must consider how she will decide whose door to knock on. If the worker is unable to visit every household, then she must consider some kind of sample.

Video

The use of video equipment may be seen as another aspect of street working but it is sufficiently distinctive in its goals and technology to be treated separately. There are few case studies from practitioners about their use of video. With the growth of neighbourhood networks on websites, blogging, mobile phones and other forms of social media, its use has probably declined. However, video can still be useful for neighbourhood workers. The following account, which also describes video's value in situations other than contact-making, is taken from a guide (no longer available) produced by Inter-Action Advisory Service.

AS AN INFORMATION TOOL At its simplest level, video can be used as a source of information about events and activities taking place in the neighbourhood. Organisations can use the equipment to produce programmes about what they are doing. This could serve either to attract more participants or members or simply to make residents aware of the kind of services or opportunities that are available, ranging from benefits and housing rights to the structure of local government. These can be played back at meetings of local groups, in the market place, in community centres or even in local pubs.

AS A 'TRIGGER' TAPE An extension of the basic information tape is the 'trigger tape' designed not only to inform people, but also to raise their level of awareness and stimulate action on any given issue. The mere presence of a group of mothers on an estate using a video camera and asking questions about the bad housing conditions will usually arouse an interest in the issue among other residents. Experience has also shown that a visual presentation of an issue rather than a verbal or written report is much more effective.

AS A WAY OF GETTING PEOPLE TO MEETINGS Video has a novelty value that will draw people to 'yet another meeting'. It is a 'telly programme' made by local people, relating directly to themselves and their neighbourhood. People come to see themselves, their kids or their neighbours on TV and, more important, they will stay on to discuss the points raised by the programme.

AS A WAY OF SHOWING COMMON PROBLEMS AND CONCERNS Video has proved instrumental in bringing both individuals and groups together by demonstrating that they share common concerns or situations. Whether it be problems of housing, education or employment, or situations common to certain groups within the community, such as children, partners or pensioners, video can be used to show that the experiences that individuals face are common problems shared by others. This process may in turn lead to a discussion of possible avenues for collective action.

AS A WAY OF ILLUSTRATING OTHER SUCCESSFUL ACTIONS On a wider scale, video can be used to link groups, geographically separate, but closely related by a common situation. Being able to show a group a tape about another group somewhere else with a similar problem, and showing the methods that were used to overcome that problem, often stimulates the viewers to attempt similar actions. As use of the Internet has demonstrated, to see that something has been done successfully elsewhere is a positive factor in the development of many groups and projects.

AS A NEW FORM OF PRESENTING INFORMATION TO AUTHORITIES Video can perform a powerful function when used in meetings with officials or experts. A videotape can often give 'ordinary' people a sense of self-confidence by putting their case in a coherent and well-thought-out form. In this way, video provides an effective voice to people who might not be given a proper hearing when other more conventional tactics such as letters, telephone calls and even delegations have failed.

AS A WAY OF EXAMINING THE DEVELOPMENT OF THE GROUP Because of its ability to provide immediate playback, video can enable a group to examine its own progress and development. Group discussions and activities can be recorded and immediately shown to the participants, either adults or children, often forcing them to analyse the way in which they react to others. This self-awareness is of benefit to both the individual and the group in that barriers to communication can be identified and dealt with.

Probes or flying kites in the community

The idea of 'probes' originated in accounts by the adult educationalist Tom Lovett of his work in Liverpool (Lovett, 1975). Probes were part of a larger strategy to make contact with local people that he describes as the exploration, investigation and experiment phase of his early work. The initiation of these probes was a reflection of the limited scope offered to the adult educator for getting in touch with parents through schools.

The probes were 'project-initiated exercises in adult education', whose purpose was both to make contacts with local people and to test their assumptions about and reactions to adult education. The probes were a project on the history of a neighbourhood run in a local school; an exhibition of the work of seven schools in a department store; and an 'informal' neighbourhood survey to 'chat people up' and discover the whole range of interests and problems.

Neighbourhood workers have used other kinds of probes such as welfare rights stalls, advice sessions, playschemes and festivals. While these provide a valuable service in their own right, they also allow the worker to enter the community in a purposive way and thus establish contact with local people. The issues or ideas around which the probes are organised may not reflect the most pressing concerns of the worker or neighbourhood – indeed, probes are valuable because these concerns may not even be known to the worker – but the probe provides a way of coming to know them.

The survey

The legitimisation of the worker's contacts is a theme that has appeared several times in this chapter, whether in regard to video, the use of leaflets when door-knocking or probes. The survey is likewise a device that legitimates the worker's activities. We have already discussed surveys and self-surveys in the chapter on data collection, and encouraged readers to refer to textbooks that will help to ensure that surveys are done with proper care and regard to the principles of social research methods. Such propriety was important because the purpose of the survey was to gather valid and reliable information on which a worker's decisions could be made. But at this stage, the worker is considering a survey primarily to make contact with people. The survey is a recruiting device and one that raises consciousness about an issue in an area. It need not, therefore, have to be so rigorous as when collecting data.

The main ways in which a contact-making survey differs from the social research kind are to do with the willingness of the worker to stay and talk with residents about issues – not just ask them questions. As a result, contacts can be built up and suspicions and mistrust towards an outsider allayed.

Surveys are also used by neighbourhood workers at the later phase of the neighbourhood process, 'forming and building an organisation', and we discuss surveys in this context in the next chapter.

The petition

Collecting signatures for a petition can serve many purposes: it can support a demand made by a local group of decision makers, gain publicity for a group and spread information about the issues with which it is concerned. It is also an aid to organising by attracting new recruits to a group, and possibly other resources such as finance. For the worker the petition is also a way into a neighbourhood in order to make contact with people and learn more about community issues. A petition carried out by the worker with one or two community residents can lead to the formation of a small group of interested people.

The small group

Most of the strategies we have discussed so far lead sooner or later to the worker meeting local residents in a small group. In one sense, then, the small group is part of these other strategies, and perhaps does not need to be treated separately. On the other hand, it represents an approach to making contacts and organising that is distinctive if only because the worker uses it to *meet* other people. The host of the group meeting will have invited residents whom the worker has not previously met. This is different from other strategies we have described when the worker meets as a group people he or she has already been in contact with individually.

The public meeting

Traditionally, the public meeting has almost always been an essential step in group development and organisation in neighbourhoods. It is through the public meeting that a constituency usually elects its committee, decides on a constitution and gives the committee a mandate from which to work. It is through the public meeting that grievances can be aired, officials confronted and the collective dimensions of a problem made manifest to individuals. It has become apparent, however, that practitioners have given less importance to the use of public meetings: they are high risk, they give residents expectations which may be unrealistic and they tend to result in existing community leaders reasserting their positions. The first two points perhaps explain the contemporary popularity of focus groups, citizens' juries, community forums and various community planning techniques. It is the last point which has led practitioners to favour networking as a key part of organising in neighbourhoods. In this section we want only to consider the public meeting *as a way of initially contacting people*, and we will leave discussion of its other functions as described earlier until the next chapter. We suggest that the points made apply also to other ways of bringing people together into some kind of public forum.

The worker using the public meeting as a contacting or recruiting mechanism will typically work by himself or herself or with some residents, using websites, emails, texting etc. and putting up posters and leaflets announcing the meeting, its agenda and where it is to be held. Such work will be preceded by a minimum of contact-making using other strategies as outlined earlier; in effect, the public meeting is called cold.

Given these circumstances, what are the factors that make for a successful public meeting? The following seem to be important, though they can all be set at nought by bad weather that persuades people to stay at home.

1   *Choose the right issue.* People will turn out if the issue is salient for them, and presented to them in a concrete and relevant way. Abstract descriptions of an issue will encourage people to stay at home; 'What's in it for me?' will be a question in many people's minds when deciding whether to turn out. 'What can *we* do about it?' is another question – the callers of the meeting will have to show some indication of the possibilities for change that can be explored if people take the first step and come to the meeting.

2   *Provide inducement to come.* Some form of entertainment is a useful inducement, as are refreshments and prize draws; so, too, is the showing of a film relevant to the issue and the presence of video and television cameras.

3   *Attend to detail in advertising and recruitment.* There should be both face-to-face contact, with residents personally invited to come and encouraged to bring friends and neighbours, as well as the use of websites, emails, posters, leaflets, networks and the media to reach a larger number of people. Reminders about the meeting are essential – leaflets should be distributed in advance of the meeting and emails sent the week of the meeting and some hours before it. If enough helpers are available people should be personally reminded through door-knocking on the

evening of the meeting, and 'fetched' to the meeting if they have expressed interest but seemed shy or diffident about attending. Another useful form of reminder is to hold a video session in the morning or afternoon, letting people know it will be shown at the meeting. Remember, too, that it can be more effective to recruit people to a meeting by going through existing networks, groups, clubs and so forth than by the 'cold' leafleting of houses and flats. Daytime meetings are more likely to be effective in neighbourhoods where residents' fear of crime inhibits their involvement in community activities after dark.

4   *Specify goals in advance.* Work out beforehand what the meeting is supposed to achieve and how this will be done. Make arrangements beforehand if you expect people to do things immediately after the meeting – it's no good asking for volunteers to put some leaflets around after the meeting if the leaflets are not available.

5   *Plan the meeting carefully.* The venue must be convenient and acceptable to most of the residents, as must the day and time of the meeting (check the television programmes and football fixtures before deciding day and time!). The size of the room is important – not so large that although there has been a good turnout it *looks* small and discourages residents; and not so small that people are uncomfortable and irritated. Seating arrangements must be thought about – arranging the audience in ranked chairs confronted by a platform of speakers is unlikely to be the most effective layout. Usually it is better to have the chairs in a semi-circle, with the table for speakers filling the gap. Work out the programme carefully, ensuring some way of keeping speakers to their time limits – and is it necessary for the meeting to spend the whole time as a large group? Finally, think about briefing 'stooges' to ask questions or to volunteer at the right time in order to get the meeting rolling.

Mediated contacts

We use the term mediated contacts to refer to those situations where some third party or event or item brings together the worker and some local residents. The fact that this occurs will often be at the initiative of the worker, so we consider it appropriate to discuss these contacts within this section.

Mediated contacts often provide, through the action of a third party, an external legitimisation both of the worker's role and interest and of his or her activity in seeking out local people to talk with them. It is not assumed, however, that this legitimisation will necessarily be helpful to the neighbourhood worker; being introduced to residents by a third party who is not well regarded may both legitimate and impair the worker's attempts to get to know local people and issues. It may also be difficult to get a conversation going with someone in the presence of a third party – perhaps the worker needs to say 'hello' casually and arrange an appointment alone with the person.

We wish to mention only some of the more common or traditional kinds of mediated contacts. These include the following:

THE GATEKEEPER OR GO-BETWEEN

The neighbourhood worker is often able to make contacts with local people through introductions made by other residents, councillors and other professionals in the neighbourhood. Each kind of go-between – whether it be a shop-keeper, regeneration officer, resident, caretaker or whoever – will carry its own costs and benefits to the worker. The worker's skill is in being able to perceive and mobilise the go-betweens that are most appropriate for each of the contacts that she or he wishes to make. To do this the worker needs some knowledge of the area, its assets and the relationships between different people and roles within it. Hence the go-between may be most safely used when the worker has begun to find her or his way around the community, and not in the early stages of intervention. People who act as go-betweens may also require something (e.g. information, support for a proposal) from the worker in return; the cost of giving this has to be accounted for when deciding whether or not to use a go-between.

GOING THROUGH EXISTING ORGANISATIONS

This way of making contacts is perhaps a special aspect of the use of a go-between. It is particularly significant in rural communities where it is all too easy for a worker to be 'frozen out' as a result of pressure from long-established organisations. Accordingly it may be a sensible practice for a worker to ask the parish council, Women's Institute or village society to introduce him. Inevitably, as with more personal go-betweens, the choice of going through one organisation rather than another pre-determines the kinds of contacts the worker will make, and the kinds of issues presented. Working through existing organisations acknowledges and respects them.

BY REFERRAL

Local people may be referred to the worker by staff in his own or other agencies. This might occur, for example, because an individual comes from the area in which it is known that the neighbourhood worker is interested, or a housing officer perceives that a client's 'problem' has a collective basis and can best be dealt with through collective action.

PUBLIC INFORMATION SOURCES

Here the worker is able to contact people through the 'mediation' of, for example, a newspaper story or a planning application. The worker might read of some named tenants in a local paper who are concerned about some aspect of their estate and take this report as an invitation to seek them out and express his interest in learning more about their concerns.

The Big Local programme, which is being run in England for Local Trust by a number of partner organisations, provides examples of mediated contacts. The programme is using advisers to support residents; the advisers will often need to make use of contacts, leaders and organisations to engage with local people (www.localtrust.org.uk).

Contacts initiated by residents

Resident-initiated contacts occur when a worker has been established in an area. He may have spent some time making contacts through ways described in the previous section, started to work with local groups and become known in the neighbourhood as a person whom people can ask for certain kinds of advice and help. As his work and interests become better known, the worker will be approached by residents and invited to discuss an issue or problem around which some local people will have already come together. Such an existing group may look to the worker for help in forming themselves into an organisation, for specific resources that they need to carry out their work more effectively or for advice on some particular aspect of their activities such as the procedures for applying to the Big Lottery Fund or the address of a partnership board chairperson.

The type of concerns that residents will thus bring to a worker will partly be determined by their perception of the worker's responsibilities and skills as they have been defined by his work with existing groups in the community; by their understanding of the remit of the worker's employing agency; and by accounts of his work and usefulness that have been disseminated along the community's informal information networks. The worker will therefore also have to negotiate misunderstandings about his role and relevance as a resource, and to respond to requests for help that are not in line with the worker's (or his agency's) priorities, skills, values and so on.

Residents will also approach a worker as a result of some event or incident in the community that brings them together or highlights a salient issue or problem. For example, unfavourable press publicity about an estate may precipitate the formation of a tenants' association or, following a road accident, parents and children may raise the issue of safe play areas.

In this part of the chapter, however, we want to deal with other kinds of resident-initiated contacts that are associated with the earlier phases of the worker's intervention. The distinguishing characteristic of this approach to contact-making is that the neighbourhood worker purposefully creates opportunities for local people to make the first contact and to take the initiative in defining an area of interest or concern. The worker 'sits back' and waits for residents to come to him; the onus is placed on residents to make use of the services that are placed at the disposal of residents, usually without much publicity and explanation. We wish in particular to examine the idea of resident-initiated contacts.

Overlapping roles

Here the worker has a role in the neighbourhood other than that of worker. He has a status or position that is additional to that of a neighbourhood worker. Perhaps the best known of overlapping neighbourhood roles is that of the worker who is also a resident in the neighbourhood in which he is working. As a consequence, the worker begins to make contact with residents, and they make contact with the worker as a resident; in this way the worker's position as a resident is one that facilitates opportunities for residents to initiate contact, sometimes relating to him as a resident, sometimes as a worker.

It is the worker–resident overlap that we want to look at further in this section, but there are also other overlaps, such as the worker who is also an employee of community group(s), and the neighbourhood worker who has another established professional role in the area such as a priest or teacher. These, too, may be seen as affording opportunities for resident-initiated contacts.

Whether one should live in the neighbourhood that one works in has been an issue of perennial discussion in community development. It is argued, on the one hand, that living in an area brings the worker familiarity with all aspects of its life, is an expression of commitment to and identification with it and provides a 'natural' way for residents to get to know the services and resources the worker can offer. It helps to overcome suspicion or distrust of outsiders and hostility to those who are perceived to commute into areas of disadvantage in order 'to do good works'. It is also suggested that residence offers one of the few ways of being responsive to events and demands in the community as they arise – problems do not confine themselves to the hours between nine and five. Neighbourhood workers will also value the satisfaction to themselves that comes of living in the neighbourhood they work in, and of being close to where the action is. Residence may be seen, too, as helping the worker to avoid importing 'outside' values and perspectives into the work in the neighbourhood.

On the other hand, it is suggested that while living in the area does have considerable benefits, it asks too much of the worker's time and energies – it increases the possibility of 'burn-out'. It blurs the boundary between work and non-work and exposes the worker to being always 'on call' to deal with group and individual problems. Besides sapping the worker of energy and interest, being on call in this way may also work against the interests of the neighbourhood. It may foster overdependence on the worker as a resource and undermine the usefulness of other local people in dealing with community issues; indeed, it may push the worker into the role of community leader. The worker is also at risk of getting too involved in neighbourhood affairs, particularly in sectional conflicts and disputes from which she should be able to distance herself in order to facilitate the work of a neighbourhood group. It is also pointed out that the family situation of some workers (e.g. a spouse tied to work in some other neighbourhood) as well as other factors like the scarcity of suitable accommodation often makes it impracticable for the worker to take up residence. A worker might also feel reluctant both to expose her family to the demands of being 'on call' and to take up living accommodation that might be needed more by other local families.

It is clear that there are arguments for and against taking up residence in a neighbourhood; our concern here is largely to point out that residence is one of the important ways in which resident-initiated contacts may be developed. Clearly, as we discussed in the previous chapter, where there are situations in which a local leader takes on the role of a neighbourhood worker, the choice facing the leader is different; by definition she lives in the area. We suspect, however, that the worker and others in this situation would do well to think through the issues we are raising in this section.

The role taken by a worker – that is, to what extent she takes up the respective roles of worker and resident – is a matter of decision in the light of factors like the characteristics of the neighbourhood and what the worker wishes to achieve. We suggest that there are three types of role:

THE RESIDENT-AS-WORKER

At this point in the continuum the person's role in the neighbourhood is mainly that of a resident. The worker might primarily *see* and identify herself as a resident first and a worker second. It is a role that can be thrust upon a worker by an event or issue that crops up in the area in which she is living. Other examples of the resident-as-worker are provided by the part-time worker who lives in the area she works in; and by the local resident who has become employed as a neighbourhood worker in the area in which she lives. Friends and neighbours may continue to relate primarily to the worker as a resident, not wanting to accept, or unable to understand, the nature of her new neighbourhood work role.

THE WORKER-AS-RESIDENT

This is the more common role, where the neighbourhood worker decides to live in the area in which she has been employed to work. The worker is probably seen primarily as an outsider whose interests and services are at first difficult to grasp, but later emerge as a helpful contribution to group activity. The worker believes that this status as a resident helps her to become better known to local people, and they are more able to understand and use her assistance. We have already discussed the pros and cons of this role.

THE COMPLETE WORKER

With this role, the neighbourhood worker does not make use of her residence in the neighbourhood to facilitate contact-making and attempts at organising. The worker may be living in the area reluctantly, and places extremely tight boundaries between her work and home and social life. The majority of the worker's contacts with local people are in the context of her neighbourhood work, and not the worker's resident role. It is perhaps difficult to imagine that this would prove to be an effective role for a neighbourhood worker. However, it might be a role that characterises the ending phase of a worker's intervention as she prepares to end work in the neighbourhood. The worker may well decide to reduce all social and non-work contacts with residents as part of her planned withdrawal. This is discussed more fully in Chapter 11 on endings in neighbourhood work.

The final point we wish to make about residence in the area of work is that the kinds of contacts that are made, and the type and quality of information gathered, will vary with particular phases of residence. This is almost a truism: the worker's contacts and information at the point of first moving into a neighbourhood are likely to be different from those when she is a firmly established resident.

Conclusions

Our purpose in this chapter has been to indicate the importance of contact-making, the functions it serves and the several forms that it may take. We are aware that, in describing the forms, we have elaborated upon methods and techniques in a way that may suggest to the reader an over-mechanistic view of the worker's tasks in making contacts with people. We accept that this may be at the cost of our presentation of the material in this chapter, but it is one that we decided to bear in order to make clear the repertoire of methods at the disposal of the worker.

We do, however, want neither to lose sight of the worker (or local people, for that matter) nor to underestimate the contributions to the success of contact-making of other, sometimes intangible, factors like the worker's stamina, enthusiasm and personal abilities to relate to a variety of individuals and groups: 'Contact with individuals and groups should always be planned, but the worker needs to be ready to utilise those unplanned, spontaneous opportunities that arise' (Smalle, personal communication).

The same point was made by one of the book's readers:

> There is something about familiarity, territory, happenstance and convenience which is important in neighbourhood work. I think lots of the formal stuff – structures, organisations, meetings – are simply vehicles or spaces for informal interaction, which then spawns other, unpredictable activities whether mutual self-help, mediating tensions and conflicts, creating/mobilising community enterprise, recruiting people, identifying and campaigning around local issues. . . . All very intangible, but vital to regeneration, social capital and social inclusion strategies.
>
> (Gilchrist, personal communication)

One of the distinctive themes in this chapter has been *choice* – choosing the kind of approach to making contacts in the light of relevant factors such as the worker's own skills and confidence, and the physical and social character of the neighbourhood. A choice has to be made in order to optimise the worker's opportunities for *communication* with local people, and the kind of communication that will help achieve greater understanding of the neighbourhood and better rapport with its residents.

We have emphasised the careful choosing and planning of the means of communication, not only to draw attention to the purposeful way in which the worker might take up the tasks of contact-making, but also to caution workers against resorting to means of contact-making without appraising those most suitable for particular circumstances. It is often too easy to turn to ways of doing things that are well tried; that one feels comfortable with; that are conveniently at hand; or that were tried 'last time'. These are sound criteria for choice only if the worker is satisfied that the methods chosen are *also* right for the situation he or she presently faces.

A feature of this chapter is its focus on the role of the neighbourhood worker. We must constantly remind ourselves that his or her actions are dependent on the energy and commitment of local people, a fundamental point illustrated by this example from a volunteer in Hungary:

> The town of Komarom is a regional centre with six secondary schools, yet ours is the only youth centre among the surrounding towns. Community places maintained by the state are not youth friendly. As parents raising youngsters, the problems affecting our children was enough for us to join forces to find a solution. That is how the decision was made: we needed to create our own community space. We bought a tiny building with a large plot of land. The house had to be re- built almost from scratch. We did it all within a year, with more than a hundred volunteers.
>
> (Eva Monostori, personal communication)

References

Alinsky, S. (1971) *Rules for radicals*, New York. Random House.

Brager, G. and Specht, H. (1973) *Community organising*, New York: Columbia University Press.

Jacobs, J. (1972) *The death and life of Great American cities*, Harmondsworth: Penguin.

Lovett, T. (1975) *Adult education, community development and the working class*, London: Ward Lock.

Rowbotham, S. (1974) *Women's consciousness, man's world*, Harmondsworth: Penguin.

Sennett, R. (2012) *Together. The rituals, pleasures and politics of co-operation*, New Haven, CT and London: Yale University Press.

Smith, M. (1994) *Local education*, Buckingham: Open University Press.

Von Hoffman, N. (1972) 'Finding and making leaders', abstracted in J. L. Ecklein and A. A. Lauffer (eds) *Community organisers and social planners*, New York: Wiley.

Wild, J. (1982) *Street mates*, Liverpool: Merseyside Youth Association.

Wilson, M. and Wilde, P. (2001) *Building practitioner strengths*, London: CDF.

7 Forming and building organisations

From group to organisation	Surveys
Community conditions	Motivations of group members
Community issues	The wider constituency
Forming an organisation	Clear goals
Checking feasibility and desirability	**Building an organisation**
Encouraging leadership	Organisational structure
Early help	Tactics and strategies
Anticipating	Group cohesion
'One thing leads to another'	**Public meetings**

> Bringing people together requires not only ability and know-how. It requires commitment, hard work and imagination – imagination to utilise the range of methods and material learnt, experimenting with combinations which will provide different ways of working, tailored to the particular issue or neighbourhood. The commitment and hard work is about never giving up. It is highly unlikely that even the most highly skilled and knowledgeable worker will get it right first time, every time.
>
> (Smalle, personal communication)

There is a rich collection of material on organising in neighbourhoods. The number of accounts of workers' successes and failures when organising groups – not all necessarily published – has grown steadily, as has the literature which describes and analyses community projects. There is good quality material in existence, most of which will be found on websites.

In our model of the neighbourhood work process, we are entering that part of practice which typically embodies the nuts and bolts of the neighbourhood worker's role. In this chapter we concentrate on the area of forming and giving strength to community groups. Then, in the following three chapters, we shall explore how to clarify goals and priorities, the business of maintaining community groups, and how they relate to other groups and organisations and provide or run services. How groups end and how workers stop supporting them is discussed in Chapter 11. This way of dividing up the formation and functioning of community groups may seem arbitrary, but we have found it to be a useful means of covering and understanding a core part of neighbourhood work practice. Inevitably, we are aware of how our generalisations cannot apply to every type of community group. We hope, however, that they are broad enough to guide the worker through the complexity of everyday practice.

DOI: 10.4324/9781003310006-7

We explore the material in this chapter under the following headings:

- From group to organisation
- Forming an organisation
- Building an organisation
- Public meetings

We attempt to identify the significant skill areas for the worker rather than provide a comprehensive analysis of existing experiences.

From group to organisation

The emphasis given by Brager and Specht (1973) to understanding *organisation building* as a distinct phase seems to us to be a helpful way of developing an analysis of community group formation. Provided one is mindful that it will usually not be easy to separate this phase from other issues and problems a group will be facing, it is a distinction we suggest is observed. It forces workers to look closely at the components which together form part of organising, rather than running them together either with the early formation of a group or with other issues an organisation faces once it has been formed.

The difference can be stated as follows: on the one hand, an informal group of individuals meeting tentatively – often emerging from a network of loosely connected people living or working in the area – to test out each other's interests, commitment and general compatibility, on the other, the deliberate formation of an organisation which has specified tasks to carry out and which has some kind of constituency and legitimacy behind it. While we continue to use the words community group within the organisation phase, we shall maintain the conceptual distinction between group and organisation, and hope to provide the reader with a credible understanding of the contrast between the two.

The substantial differences between a fledgling community group and a group which has clear organisational characteristics often receive only limited attention from both workers and groups. The central question is: how will this grouping of individuals hold together once it changes from being an informal, often temporary group to a more public and possibly permanent organisation? Will the same people, for example, wish to participate, or will the formation of an organisation require a different set of capacities and skills from those used in a group?

The worker needs to help group members check out that they do in fact share approximately the same understanding and opinion about a problem or issue. It is essential for them to have an awareness of what they are taking on when they shift from being part of a group to an organisation. There has accumulated sufficient experience in neighbourhood work for practitioners to speak with confidence on this point: involvement of local people over and above their other commitments can take a heavy toll on domestic and social life. A neighbourhood worker who is working closely with an active, busy group will be meeting one or more of its members daily, while the members will be engaged in carrying out a range of successive tasks. In addition, they will naturally be drawn into informal discussion among themselves about the group, and talk with neighbours, friends and relatives about their work, often trying to encourage them to join in.

All this consumes the time and energy of people who will often have partners and families to support and who will face a variety of economic pressures. Some community leaders who are representatives on partnership boards reckon to spend about 20 hours a week working on behalf of their communities. This may be unusually high, but the general point about the implication of individuals committing themselves to playing an active part in community activities, and the effects of this on private lives, is applicable to most active community groups. An understanding of some of the possible costs, as well as the benefits, of being involved in a group can be fostered by a neighbourhood worker as individuals move from being part of a loose, informal grouping to becoming members of an organisation. The contrast between networks and organisations is discussed by Alison Gilchrist: 'Organisations use rules to coordinate activity. Networks need relationships to influence behaviour and change minds' (Gilchrist, 2019: 34).

Inevitably, the process of forming a community group, and the tasks involved, will vary considerably according to local circumstances. Two important variables will be the extent of social interaction and community activity existing already in a neighbourhood, and the nature of the issue around which a group of people forms. The two variables are relevant whatever the predisposition of the worker, and we shall examine each in turn.

Community conditions

What degrees of energy and apathy exist in different kinds of neighbourhoods? What do we mean by a 'strong' community and by 'apathy' and how can each of them be recognised? These questions point to problems facing a neighbourhood worker, especially when residents appear to have little contact with each other and when the worker knows very few people. The importance of how local people perceive their community, and how they think outsiders perceive it, can never be underestimated. A study of two estates in Middlesbrough and Stockton found that:

> Residents felt stigmatised because they lived in estates with a poor reputation. They believed people living outside the estates thought they were criminals and that their children were out of control. This unwanted stereotyping was deeply resented.
>
> (Joseph Rowntree Foundation, 1999: 2)

Such feelings have, in our opinion, become more widespread in the years subsequent to this study.

Analysis of community conditions is of critical importance for regeneration programmes committed to supporting sustainable communities. The research, referred to in Chapter 1, showing the existence of the community sector also showed that a proportion of residents in all areas are involved in local public life:

> Autonomous local activity takes place at many levels and in varying degrees. The most sustained form of involvement is through local community organisations or groups, ranging from small informal groups meeting in people's homes or in public places to well-established voluntary organisations with their own premises and staff.
>
> (Chanan, 1997: 9)

The findings of this and subsequent research are a useful source for community development and regeneration programmes. Neighbourhood workers still have to undertake their own audits and analyses of neighbourhoods but, over the last decade, researchers have created a knowledge bank to which practitioners and managers can turn.

Participation in community affairs can challenge the negative stereotypes which outsiders hold of communities, and set in motion a positive cycle. The beginning of such changes is usually at a small and modest level where the activity strikes chords in enough individuals to make them want to come together, and to stay together as a collective unit.

A significant theme in community development is the extent to which neighbourhoods and groups of people who are considered to be apathetic, unenterprising or depressed can demonstrate the vigour, initiative and skills which in fact exist in them. Neighbourhood work speaks to the strengths of communities. The willingness to be involved may need sparking, and this can be done as a result of a threat or a problem (a gang culture, a main road planned to come through an estate, vandalism etc.), through the energies of community leaders, or by the intervention of a neighbourhood worker; often it is a combination of all three. The experiences of working with unorganised or poorly organised groups of employees have driven home the same point, as the London Living Wage campaigns launched in 2001 and organised by Citizens UK, demonstrated: low-paid shift workers, home-workers, night office cleaners and other exploited groups have benefits of mutual support, as well as improvements in their conditions, through the efforts they made to organise themselves. In doing so they raised their own self-esteem and demonstrated their resourcefulness to others.

Neighbourhood workers are constantly looking for signs of interest and activity in communities which they can help to foster. By training and inclination they are motivated towards nosing out concerns in a neighbourhood which are amenable to being debated and supported on a community basis. They are, in effect, in business to 'pick up' on issues which may be dormant in a community. This perspective may lead them to be relatively optimistic about the potential for action lying in so-called apathetic communities.

Neighbourhood workers certainly need to become skilled at utilising existing informal networks of support and activity in neighbourhoods as well as capitalising on existing leadership. In the literature on old industrial communities (mining, steel, docking or shipbuilding areas), it is pointed out that many community projects benefited from the history of collective industrial action, making active organising by the community more likely to develop. The fallacy is to transfer such conditions and activity to other communities seemingly facing similar problems. The process of understanding about a community and its history (as discussed in Chapter 4) has to precede the borrowing of organising strategies and tactics tried elsewhere; it cannot be seen as an afterthought or as being of a secondary order to the business of working with community groups.

It would seem that there must be a tension between the neighbourhood worker's role as an agent of change, a facilitator, enabler and organiser, and the need to respect the existing fabric of the community where he or she works. It is one thing for the worker to have an adequate knowledge of the sociology of communities; it is another to apply it in practice to specific communities.

Awareness of the different levels of community leadership, and their degrees of formality and informality, needs to be part of workers' assessment. How they identify the different levels, and how and when they seek to get them interacting, remain questions, which continually test workers' skills and judgement.

Community issues

We turn now to our second variable influencing the transformation of an informal grouping of individuals to an organisation: the nature of the issue or concern which may bind them together and lead them to some kind of common commitment. The seedbed for such a growth of awareness, and the time it takes for awareness to lead to organisation, naturally will depend on whether the issue arises out of debate within a small informal network, at one extreme, or out of a national or international social movement, at the other. These are polar extremes, and in between them there lies an infinite combination of possibilities, most of them involving, at any one time, national, regional and local factors.

Most issues around which people form are very localised and do not link directly to city-wide or national debates. The realisation, for example, in a community of the value of starting a good neighbourhood scheme for older people grows out of local people's own awareness of the need and what they can do about it. The influence of outside factors, such as promotion by Age UK or a policy statement by a government department, remains marginal.

Clearly related to whether an issue is predominantly local or national in origin is the question of its content. A worker who is going to 'run with an issue', with the aim of gathering support, stands a good chance if it has to do with housing, the environment, jobs, library closures or play. Concerns that appear not to generate the same degree of immediate support might be a drugs prevention project, the need for teenage facilities and community care schemes for older people. Health issues may lie somewhere between the two: a hospital threatened with closure can mobilise community opposition rapidly; so too can health hazards to an entire community. Less dramatically, the connections between health improvement, regeneration and community development have strengthened significantly in recent years.

The aforementioned examples of the content of issues, and the broad divisions we have made, are generalisations. We underline their relevance, however, to neighbourhood workers who are in the position of judging when and with what expectations they should assist with the formation of a community group. They can be helped in this critical area by drawing upon guidelines, based upon experience, about the local–national focus of the issue or concern and about its content.

The worker can also make use of a more abstract framework. This can be portrayed as a scale, which includes the decision of local people to form a group because they feel themselves to be under some threat, and the formation of a group because a number of people perceive an opportunity and decide to take it. It can be extended or made more sophisticated but may provide some guidance about the formation of groups (see Table 7.1).

In focusing on the relevance of community conditions and issues, we have not attempted to answer the question of why community groups do spring up. Rather, we have isolated two factors which influence the decision of a group to give itself an organisational form. Clearly there will be wide variation in the steps which groups of individuals take and the length of time involved in each part of the organising process. It will depend, not least, on the kind of organisation which is being created – a youth work project, a residents' association, an environmental project, a development trust – each will inevitably make different demands on people's organising capacities and will need particular organisational arrangements.

Forming and building an organisation cannot follow any kind of blueprint. Yet it may be that a worker can offer invaluable help and advice to a group through his or her ability to separate out some of the relevant community conditions from the real or potential issues facing a group of individuals. A study of two estates in Bradford underlines the extent to which many residents not only experience fear and insecurity but also have strong prejudices and resentments, echoing society and the media's view of them as 'other' – that is 'different' and 'lower':

> Prejudice and resentment could be expressed towards people from other commu-
> nity centres and organisations, those living in different 'territories' on the estate,
> those with mental health issues, 'problem families' or newcomers. Tensions were
> highest on the smaller estate, which already had a significant proportion of British
> Asian households and more recently Slovakian and Slovakian-Roma families and
> some asylum seekers. Conflicts flared occasionally and could take violent forms.
> (Joseph Rowntree Foundation, 2010: 2–3)

Neighbourhood workers can help communities facing such complex social conditions to separate out the imagined issues from the real ones and encourage people to focus on the latter.

The nature of particular communities and the range of possible issues which could bring benefits to them are tightly bound together. It is a worker's task to be aware of

Table 7.1 A framework for group formation

Theme	Why groups form	Examples of organising issues
Threat	External threat	Major road planned through high density housing area
	Intra-community threat	School closure
	Inter-communal tension	Asian and white people in London's East End
	Failure of power holders	Inadequate repairs
	Response to an action perceived as unfair	Rent increases
	Hazards for residents	Child falls from balcony
Opportunity	New resources	Community centre
	Significant change in composition of neighbourhood	Regeneration
	Change of political party in control of local authority	New policy on community centres
	Groups in other neighbourhood are perceived to obtain success	Installation of CCT

this and to point out to those with whom he is working some of the difficulties they face in this respect – at a point when they are open to his advice, and when the worker judges that he could offer his understanding of their communities and the issues which could bring them together. Such general advice can complement work done on particular details of a group's formation. The importance of the worker deciding when to intervene in this way will become clearer in the following section, which analyses the range of possible tasks to be completed during the phase of helping the formation of an organisation.

Forming an organisation

The job of organising in a neighbourhood can accommodate most kinds of worker style or character. Quiet determination, for example, can be as effective as extrovert charisma. The important 'mix' is between the personal qualities and strengths of a worker and his or her ability to maintain an awareness of the tasks which need to be undertaken – particularly as the organising becomes more hectic and demanding.

We suggest that, rather than good organising being seen to derive almost entirely from 'secret' or natural talents, as much effort as possible should be given to making organising skills explicit.

We propose to offer such an explication, first by setting out six points a worker can refer to when organising, and then by offering three general guidelines. The six points are checking feasibility and desirability, encouraging leadership, early help, anticipating, 'one thing leaders to another', and surveys.

Checking feasibility and desirability

Neighbourhood workers rightly seek to remain close to their major brief: to help form community groups and encourage and support them to take action. Their motivation and terms of employment focus on working with collectivities. Local people who are in contact with neighbourhood workers mostly have similar expectations. Yet forming a group is not necessarily or automatically always in the best interest of a particular collection of individuals. We have referred already to the internal strain group organising can create on participants. Other factors to watch out for are the following:

Existing groups

A group or organisation may already exist in the *same* area, and the worker may be confident that it can meet the needs of a group of individuals who are considering forming a new organisation. Why duplicate? The worker may often be in a position to advise because people may only be half aware of an existing organisation, or not really believe one exists. This can happen on a large estate, especially when there is a high rate of mobility. Clearly the worker has to balance advice she gives about other relevant organisations with her understanding of some of the covert reasons why a group of people may want to start a new group (rivalry, personality conflict, status). The worker must also give due weight to one of the canons of community development theory: if people want to act together they have the right to do so; otherwise, phrases about people expressing their own needs, unabetted and without interference, take on a hollow ring.

Neighbouring groups

Equally, a similar organisation to the one being proposed may exist already in a *nearby* area. Would there be better pay-offs for both areas if interest and commitment within them were harnessed to one organisation? There could be benefits in keeping to one organisation which has sufficiently broad goals to encompass more than one set of interests; the common aims of each area might be achieved more swiftly and effectively. Examples can be found in regeneration areas facing similar problems or fighting for the same solutions; street groups can be more effective in one consolidated group or forum than if they each set up on their own, although this should not imply that workers should not organise on a street basis.

Potential membership

The likely membership of a proposed organisation may be small. If a neighbourhood worker, as a result of their experience and ability to analyse a situation, is convinced of this, why allow a group of people to move ahead under the illusion that active support will snowball? Failure, under these circumstances, would be inevitable and often destructive. A worker who thinks she can prevent this happening need have no qualms about advising the group to hold back from starting an organisation. In case this appears to put too much power in the hands of the worker, we again emphasise the importance of leaving decisions in the end to those involved.

Timing

It may not be an appropriate time for an informal group to move into an organisational phase. The members may not be strong enough as a collective, the situation around which they propose to organise may not be sufficiently clear, it may be important to wait upon the outcome of one or more external factors. There could be a number of reasons, in other words, why a worker might say in effect to a group, 'I am fully behind you, and I think what you are doing is right, but my advice is to wait a bit'.

Thinking about strategy

Finally, it is conceivable that the strategy of forming an organisation may in itself be a weak one, regardless of its timing. It may be, for example, that the last action a worker should encourage among young people on an estate where hostility to young people from adults is bitter would be the creation of a youth action group – not necessarily because of the worker's anxieties about escalation of conflict but in order not to worsen the lives of the young people themselves. Or, in an area of unemployment, it may be more relevant to concentrate energies on supporting existing organisations rather than attempt to set up a new one – there may, for example, be a resource centre which offers a base for taking action to deal with the effects of public expenditure cuts and unemployment in the community, helping benefit claims, for example, reducing boredom and frustration, or harnessing anger.

These two examples are given to emphasise the point that there need be no reverence for community groups as being good in themselves. Examining possible alternative or complementary approaches before making a commitment to organise can be a healthy means of checking on the feasibility and desirability of establishing community groups. It can also make for stronger organising.

Encouraging leadership

Searching out and supporting individuals who can become leaders of community groups are crucial in neighbourhood organising. The growth in the number of social entrepreneurs adds a complication because their approach tends to favour strong leadership; neighbourhood workers and regeneration officers are looking for this quality in potential entrepreneurs. Caution, however, in moving too quickly to identify community leaders is advisable.

> A common mistake made in neighbourhood consultation and involvement strategies is consistently to only include the well-known people, organisations and groups. All too often those who shout the loudest, and who already have the ears of lead officers and funders, are the sections of the neighbourhood contacted. Rudimentary networks are developed, resulting in exclusive rather than inclusive involvement.
>
> (Smale, personal communication)

The identification of local leadership is usually a difficult task for a worker, and full of uncertainty. Much of her time will be spent in talking individually with those who have expressed an interest in taking on leadership roles – chairperson, secretary, convenor, treasurer of a group, or simply being on the organising committee.

The worker will wish to work through with each of them the duties involved when taking on a leadership position, what the commitment will imply in terms of time and energy, and how the assumptions of a leadership role will be viewed by other members of the group. At the same time, the worker will be trying to decide whether a particular person or persons will make effective leaders: Von Hoffman's warnings about plucking out 'natural leaders' have been referred to already (Chapter 6); wrong choices can mean early disaster for a group.

We shall see later that the element of uncertainty in encouraging leadership has implications for the early structuring of organisations. What, though, does the worker look for when wanting to encourage leadership within an emerging group? It is impossible to offer firm guidelines, or a checklist, of leadership qualities. It would, however, seem important that individuals can:

- demonstrate real commitment to the purpose of the group they will be involved with;
- feel confident that they can take on a leadership role;
- show they are aware of the need to hold the trust and support of the group, in situations which will sometimes test their stamina and loyalty;
- be committed to democratic forms of organising and to involving others;
- be aware of the amount of time that will be required of a leader.

These are just five relevant qualities for a leader of most types of community groups. The positive qualities which a potential community leader possesses can be the ones which cause difficulty later on – great forcefulness, strongly held convictions, for example. A worker will often greatly influence a group's choice of leaders by actions such as with whom she leaves messages and whose house she calls at – or who she does not contact. The latter may be held against her later.

> There is an old saying from the Caribbean which became clear to me as a neighbourhood worker – 'Late invitation suit fools'. Time and again, members of the neighbourhood would repeat this to me, usually when contact was initiated, in their minds, either as an afterthought or rather late in the day.
>
> (Smalle, personal communication)

It is essential to continue to search out new leadership, and workers should avoid the temptation to go for 'safe' or existing leaders in the community when they are involved in helping to organise a group. Neighbourhood work tries to reach those without power, authority or status, sometimes groups which are stigmatised by the rest of society. Leadership must come from within the groups themselves as well as from outside them.

More pragmatically, the choice or acceptance of a leader who already has some leadership role or status in the community can defeat the very purpose of organising, because people in a group will tend to feel that he or she cannot give a full commitment to it. Consequently their own investment in it will dwindle. In taking this view we do not wish to suggest that elected members, religious leaders, youth workers and others should never become leaders of community groups. We are offering, rather, a general principle for this key aspect of organising against which a worker can compare particular practice situations. It is certainly unwise, if not disingenuous, for workers to underestimate the amount of influence they can bring to bear on the process involved in choosing leaders. Given the evidence that exists of the work pressures that community representatives on partnership boards and forums experience, the need for workers to advise likely leaders of what lies in store for them has considerable importance.

In addition to the time to be put in by the worker when encouraging individuals to think about and decide upon taking up leadership positions, there is the value such meetings can have for the individuals concerned. A worker is often welcomed into people's homes to discuss the hopes and fears for an emerging community group. At other times the worker will be involved in what may seem to be continuous hospitality in cafés and community centres, picking up key remarks made about forming an organisation and being introduced to new faces who could become future members of the group the worker is concerned with. The worker will also aim to increase the confidence of individuals at group meetings. The objective, in each instance, is for the worker to transmit her skills so that a group can take on increasing responsibilities and become more than a loose collection of like-minded people.

The period between a decision in principle of a group of people to organise themselves properly, often represented by the setting up of a steering committee, and the fruition of the decision, can be exhausting and depressing for group members. In addition, it not only provides opportunities for a worker to be extremely active, because of their knowledge and experience of how other groups have handled this situation, but it also requires the worker to be very open with group members as a person. The development of 'warm informal relationships' with individuals can make it easier for the worker's advice to be acceptable. More important, it can begin to assure people of the worker's willingness to go along with them.

Our own and others' experience points, therefore, to the need for closeness and reciprocity between worker and group members, especially potential leaders, at this stage. The amount of time and energy involved in this kind of work, most of it outside any formal or public setting, is often underestimated by both practitioners and their employing agencies.

Early help

We have deliberately separated the question of whether or not a worker takes a leadership role from the earlier discussion of leadership. Neighbourhood work seeks to encourage local leadership; it has as an implicit aims the devolving of existing sources of power – including that of the neighbourhood worker – in the belief that increased awareness and control by local people over a range of decisions have intrinsic value. *How* such a process is facilitated is another matter, but doubtless both directive and non-directive workers would agree on the aforementioned objective.

It may be that even the worker most committed to the non-directive approach may see it as both relevant and justifiable for him or her to assume some kind of leadership role in the formation phase of a community group. Leadership as a useful method of working with a group in the early stages of its formation can, in this sense, be distinguished from objectives and values concerning indigenous leadership.

Alinsky recounts a cautionary tale of how too much expertise and self-confidence by a worker can reinforce people's doubts about their own capacities and stop them from taking the first steps to organising. To themselves, the people of Muddy Flats thought:

> 'That smart New Yorker must certainly think I'm dumb – I've lived here for forty years in all of this mess and that smart guy has to come around to tell me why I've been living in all this mess. What he's really saying when he tells me that I should come to that Friday night meeting is that I'm too dumb to know enough to do something about it. So if I go to the meeting I'm really admitting to him, and certainly to myself, that I am dumb.' So he doesn't go.
>
> (Alinsky, 1969)

We are wary of introducing the notion of the worker becoming a leader – albeit a temporary one – of a group, or assuming a leadership role, because it puts so much onto the worker. Forming a community group does imply members taking some risks, and these cannot and should not be eliminated by the worker becoming a leader of the group.

A worker who does so is likely to store up problems for the group in the future, because she or he is placing them in a false cocoon. Sooner or later, when the worker may no longer be around, the group will become exposed and vulnerable to internal and external pressures, and it needs to be prepared for them. The worker should therefore resist temptations and pressures to take on a major leadership role which should be filled by a member of the group, despite the difficulties at times of doing so.

However, if the risks facing those who are forming a group cannot be eliminated, they can certainly be minimised by a neighbourhood worker. This suggests a different mode of leadership, and essentially takes the form of the worker offering services and help to the group, often in a direct and concrete way. They can be offered on a scale and with a degree of intensity at this point of the organising process so as to be able to contrast it with later phases, when help of the kind to which we are referring would certainly be misplaced. We suggest, in short, that there is value in a worker taking on a quasi-leadership role temporarily.

The most common form of early help provided by a worker is the carrying out of a plethora of small tasks. It could mean taking an active part in the planning and implementing of an initial fund-raising event for a group, such as a jumble sale: booking the hall, organising the collection of items, obtaining and setting up tables, ensuring a rota of helpers, helping clear up afterwards. The worker's active participation in such tasks may have a twofold function: showing people *how* to do certain things, such as booking a school hall through the local education authority and the head of the school, and demonstrating their personal commitment to the group's future. Despite connotations of condescension, the deliberate involvement of the worker in a group's early activities and her willingness to carry messages on its behalf is important and justified.

It goes without saying that the occasion and opportunity for this type of intervention by the worker will vary greatly. Some groups will have enough skill, knowledge, instinct and confidence to do without the worker; frequently they will be in the position of teaching her. Yet we suggest that many will not, and will benefit considerably from having the active support of a worker. What is important, when undertaking a succession of tasks, is for the worker to remember her educator role, passing on skills and knowledge, enhancing the capacity of group members to be heard, to hear, understand and participate.

Sometimes it is helpful for a worker to inform a group which is organising about groups similar to itself and to suggest one or more visits. The groups might be at different stages of development, thereby enabling the visiting group members to have their ambitions and plans both reaffirmed and challenged. The visits need not be limited to the area within which the group is located; for example, a group of people proposing to start a community transport scheme in Stepney went to Liverpool to see such a scheme in operation, in addition to visiting schemes in other parts of London. Naturally, the ability of a worker to offer this and other kinds of specific, task-focused help depends on her having sufficient basic knowledge of the availability of resources, and of how to find out about opportunities and resources quickly. Awareness of the level and accessibility of resources required are perhaps the key to the ability of the worker to offer direct help, and to run errands for a group as it moves towards becoming an organisation.

Anticipating

A more reflective task, which complements the sense of activity suggested by the provision of direct aid, has to do with the need to look ahead. What major problems or blockages is a group likely to meet and what should a worker who is confident of his forecast do? Should the worker present his viewpoint to the group and thereby try to persuade it to change its approach, or should the worker leave it to continue, and possibly make damaging mistakes? An example will illustrate the dilemma we are pointing to:

> A group of tenants in a block of flats starts to meet twice weekly and plans to form a tenants' association. A neighbourhood worker is invited to the meetings, but he feels there is limited scope for him to intervene: it is a group with too many ideas. Individuals put forward one idea after the other. Someone agrees to write them down but it is not made clear in what capacity he does so. The ideas range from projects (a cleaning rota for the lifts, outings for older people, a playscheme, a visit to the seaside), to fund-raising (a fete, a lottery, an art competition, a sponsored swim) to political strategy (attending area forum meetings, requesting officers of the local authority to attend one of their meetings, lobbying councillors).
>
> The stream of ideas sounds to the worker more appropriate for a strong, well-organised association which has gained some experience, rather than for a newly emerging group. He anticipates that few if any of the ideas will be put into action; individuals will become disillusioned and the early organisation of the tenants will break apart. Should the worker warn the group that this is likely to happen? How can he do this without blunting enthusiasm or appearing as a 'know-all' and risking making himself rather than the group the focal point of the initiative?

The example illustrates how workers have to develop different group work skills in order to handle the various stages of a group's growth; in this instance how to warn the group of the likely consequences of its lack of internal control without dampening the all-important initial drive of a group. A worker's relationship with group members in this kind of situation, the skills the worker displays to them and the role he adopts will contrast with the worker's relationships once the group has formed. Many of the skills will focus on acting as a clarifier of others' contributions in a meeting, amplifying them, and translating them into other terms if they are misunderstood. The worker can spell out some of the consequences of various points put forward, leaving the meeting to decide what action should be taken.

Similarly, the worker should not hold back from anticipating external problems that a group may face, as when an inexperienced group is vulnerable to being co-opted or sucked in by an existing organisation, leading to the loss of an important element of autonomy. We think the worker has a responsibility to alert a disorganised group to this possibility and spell out what the effects might be.

'One thing leads to another'

Neighbourhood workers often carry in their minds the thought that out of the formation of one group, others will emerge.

There is nothing sinister about this. The awareness that new activities are likely to spring out of first initiatives reflects our knowledge of how and why people decide to join organisations and make them viable. If a worker were to misuse this knowledge, by abandoning or even sabotaging a group they had helped to form, or by unilaterally giving all their allegiance to other groups in the locality, evidently this would be a form of manipulation and should be deplored. In our experience few workers act in this way. It would run counter to the strongly held value in neighbourhood work of encouraging a multiplicity of activities, of always encouraging systems to remain 'open'.

The awareness that small beginnings may lead to further community organising can be used by a worker helpfully and creatively. Generally, it can take two forms: a group may itself turn into either an extended or a different kind of organisation, or the formation of one group may stimulate the growth of others around related issues or common interests. In our experience, both of these patterns are likely to occur in neighbourhoods which are generally poorly resourced. When people see neighbours making progress on a particular issue, their confidence increases to a point where they decide to take action on other needs in the community.

The notion of one thing leading to another can be applied to a range of activities. It may be particularly relevant to activities which people really enjoy doing: the creative, celebratory, 'fun element' in neighbourhood work should never be underestimated. In addition to being valuable in itself, it can also lead to other forms of action. There are often an important links between community art and neighbourhood work.

We suggest that the notion of a creative dynamic between one activity and others need not remain simply a haphazard possibility but may be thought about by the neighbourhood worker and shared with people they are working with. This approach needs to be combined with the realisation that new initiatives will happen unexpectedly, reflecting the interest and energies of a group or network at a particular time. This point is made by Anne Sloman in her discussion of participatory theatre in community development: 'When used well, it builds community cohesion and can help communities address issues. It can be a celebration for peace and fun, while it also has the flexibility to explore any number of areas' (Sloman, 2012: 55).

Surveys

Neighbourhood workers make use of surveys to assist communities to organise, and we have discussed them in Chapters 4 and 6. They can also be used alongside a number of other actions within an *integrated* strategy aimed at stimulating and encouraging organisation at a local level. The use of street representatives, and the holding of a public meeting, can be essential ingredients of the use of the survey. It can work primarily as a neighbourhood work intervention and, second, as an information-gathering instrument. Workers may be familiar with the experience of using a survey of a neighbourhood: they obtain a very poor response and very little information. Then the few people who showed interest come together. They re-word the questionnaire, organise the survey and collect useful information. That can be the beginning of a group.

Other techniques which can often be used in conjunction with a survey are video and a petition. The former can support a survey's findings with visual evidence and the voices of the people affected by a particular problem. The latter can be an effective means of capitalising on the results of a survey. People can be presented with hard information about their area or an issue and thereby be in a position to see the relevance of signing a petition. The wish to take action may be particularly strong if there has been a high involvement of local people in the survey.

The danger of raising too high expectations of action through use of the survey should be noted. It can lead to disillusionment about organising. This points to the importance of clear thinking and detailed planning about how to make use of a survey as a means of forming a community organisation.

We have drawn attention to six categories of skill areas in the initial organising phase of neighbourhood work. There will be many others which workers draw upon; equally, those which we have highlighted will be applied in other phases of community groups too. Before we examine the tasks facing the worker when building an organisation, we shall end our discussion of the formation phase with three general comments.

Motivations of group members

First, a statement of the obvious: people give time and energy to community groups for a variety of private and public reasons. Motivations and aspirations of individuals inevitably influence the direction of an emerging group and the speed and ease with which it will become an organisation. People may first have to meet their own personal needs before they can solve the problems of others and of the community; or such a stance may be rejected, and the thrust will be to help people make connections between their private ills and public problems. It is not within our brief to open this debate here. We wish merely to draw attention to the need for neighbourhood workers to remain aware of the degree to which motivations of group members are likely to differ, and for them to be able to respond to personal interests and demands within group or collective contexts. It takes us back to the concept of social capital, which we discussed in the introductory chapter, and the degree of risk that poor people may take when deciding whether or not to participate in a community group.

We still do not have a full understanding of why poor neighbourhoods do not always organise spontaneously or easily. It requires careful analysis of why people do and do not become involved in different environments and under particular conditions. The benefits for neighbourhood workers of this knowledge would lie in their increased ability to respond to the priorities and interests of local people.

The wider constituency

Evidence that a group of individuals is set upon forming itself into an organisation will draw a neighbourhood worker, who may be in uncertain contact with it, into an initial working relationship. We have seen that the worker will wish to be identified with the efforts of group members, and that he will become involved in undertaking tasks for them. While the worker does these things, he needs, as it were, to keep glancing over his shoulder at the wider community. Above all, the worker needs to retain the group's awareness of its wider constituency. In the example of the Silvertop estate in Antwerp, the tenants' group is clear that it is acting on behalf of other residents of the tower blocks, many of whom are not Belgian:

> Representation is not, according to the community development worker, the first issue in the tenants' participation. It is much more important that there is an active group of occupants which is prepared to take responsibility for the project and which gives others the opportunity to participate. . . . The actual tenant's

group consists of a more or less stable nucleus of twenty-five people, which can be widened depending on the activities or issues.

(Hautekeur, personal communication)

A similar concern should inform action in an area divided between old-established residents and newcomers, where the latter are often scapegoated by the former for the area's deterioration. A continuing feedback process can be very important in these situations.

In its concern to organise itself, a community group can easily lose sight of the need and value of keeping in touch with neighbours who are not involved and with other local groups, both of whom may be affected by the group's subsequent action. Equally, in the situation where a group has come together with great difficulty and is very unsure of itself, it can be important for it to show the neighbourhood that it is alive and functioning by organising an event or activity early on – an outing for older people, a playscheme, even a brief report delivered to every household. None of these may fit the central purpose of the group, but by doing them the group may both help the necessary climate of opinion and retain its constituency. It will then be in a better position to continue and grow as an organisation. If the group concentrates solely on its own meetings – planning, discussing and developing – it will be perceived as inward-looking or as a paper organisation by others because there is nothing to convince them otherwise. In the long run, such early negative attitudes are likely to rebound on the group.

Clear goals

Goals and objectives of a group which at the beginning seemed reasonably clear if not self-evident often start to appear complex, confused and elusive as time goes on. The worker has a vital role to play in helping a group to clarify its aims, and in ensuring that a period or mood of confusion does not continue. As new ideas emerge about how to tackle a particular issue, and as new members join the group, aims will naturally change. Again, the worker needs to be aware of shifts in attitude or position, of changes in aspiration and strategy, and work on them with the group. We shall see that this forms a key part of both building and maintaining an organisation.

The work at the early part, however, is equally important and may require the worker to be challenging, critical and provocative towards a group if he or she thinks its aims are unclear, woolly or over-ambitious. The worker needs, in effect, to be putting to the group the questions: 'What are you in business for? What are you trying to do?' 'As well as your overall aims, what are your specific objectives?' Clarity and agreement will enable the group to work better on key questions such as membership, funds, timing and structures.

A worker should help a group to be as precise as possible as to what it is trying to do before it moves too rapidly into an action-oriented and consolidating phase. By then there will be a number of other tasks to undertake, and it is well for them to be informed by clarity of aims. The contribution of the worker on this point represents the keynote to the formation of effective community groups. Evidently there is a clear link between work done on clarifying goals and setting priorities once a group is established (see Chapter 8).

Encouraging a group to be clear about its aims and objectives needs to be undertaken with an awareness that, in the early stages, group members will be getting to know each other. Time should be planned for people to talk informally and check out those things which have been discussed more formally.

Building an organisation

Building community organisations calls upon the abilities of workers and leaders to make judgements about *when* to act and *what* to introduce; every group will require a unique combination of organisational, professional, political and emotional support.

The period between the first early meetings of a group and the time when action begins to flow from the work and strength of the group is of paramount importance. There may be relatively little to show for it externally, yet it is the period when the foundations of an effective local organisation are laid. There will be many decisions to make and tasks to undertake. There will also need to be work done on the internal, interactional functioning of a group. We propose to examine these questions by concentrating on the following three areas:

- Organisational structure
- Tactics and strategies
- Group cohesion

Organisational structure

The question of how organised a group should be needs to be near the top of the neighbourhood worker's agenda. How structured and formal should a group be? It is a question, it should be remembered, which is relevant for all phases of the existence of a community group, because organisational requirements are likely to change as the nature and purpose of the group change. Cary has suggested that community organisations tend to develop through at least three stages: the initial stage of organisation, the task accomplishment stage and the stage of continuity or discontinuity. We are concerned at this point with the first of these. It is a time which places great demands on leaders: 'Persons with ideas and the ability to implement ideas contribute heavily during this initial stage' (Cary, 1970).

Differences between kinds of community groups assume particular importance now. They increase the difficulty of generalising about organisational structure. The following nine types, based on the experiences of Community Development Foundation projects, suggest the range and variety of groups:

Self-help groups: Those which are run by the people who benefit from them, such as food cooperatives or playgroups.

User groups: Those which are run by people using a service, such as people with learning disabilities.

Care groups: Those which provide a service for other people, such as good neighbour schemes.

Representative groups: Elected by and answerable to the community – tenants' and residents' associations are obvious examples.

Minority interest groups: Groups that aim to improve the rights of certain sections of the population; examples are single parents' and black groups.

Issue groups: These consist of people committed to taking action on particular topics, such as the local economy, the environment or children's safety. They can be self-appointed or representative and they take action in what they see to be the interests of the whole community. They will include social enterprise groups.

Community forums: These, arguably, are only partly community groups as they are set up for debate and decision-making among a number of groups.

Traditional organisations: Well-established groups, usually catering for a particular sector of the community, such as women's institutes and working men's clubs.

Volunteer groups: People who commit themselves to take care of public amenities such as parks and woodlands.

Social groups: Those which exist solely to put on social events; they range from loose groups of neighbours who organise trips to quite large festival committees, sports leagues and associations for various hobbies.

These are approximate definitions of the different types of community group. Many will fall into more than one category, and a further type could be added – that of identity, political and other groups characterised by having a philosophy by which they analyse a neighbourhood's problems and from which they find their strength. They may also be able to call on outside support for resources and for maintaining groups. Examples range from faith groups to socialists, environmentalists, pacifists, secret societies and political parties.

The typology helps us to appreciate how the organisational structure which is developed needs, above all, to be related to the functions it is going to play. Baldock (1974) argues that this factor is more important than that of the manner in which the group came together in determining the degree of formality or informality of structure.

We shall return to the question of formal and informal organisation after referring to four related issues which can be usefully differentiated in a discussion of the organisational structure of community groups.

Membership

Most groups will start with a few people, and they will immediately be concerned with encouraging others to join them. The prior question, however, needs to be, 'Why do you want members anyway?' The question is asked in order to encourage groups to be explicit about the advantages of having a large membership and to guide them in making effective use of members. It should not be assumed that membership is a good thing in itself. The following are some of the benefits: the more people involved in the group the more activities it can undertake; the more it can be aware of the issues that concern and interest people, the more it can be seen as representative; the stronger it is to undertake collective action, the more effectively it can relate to partnerships, local agencies and voluntary organisations. Greater fund-raising potential and a larger pool of skills and human resources to draw upon can also be advantageous. The popularity of crowd funding is a good illustration. Yet there can be no firm guidelines about the size of a group; too many members with no sense of real attachment to the group can be as damaging as too few.

As important as the number of members are the problems of staying in touch with existing members and recruiting new ones. The first requires a two-pronged strategy: first, ensure that as many people as possible are involved at different levels of a group's activities; second, make certain that there is good communication within the group: a regular newsletter if membership is large; reports of executive and other committee meetings. Such written or electronic methods can be complemented by encouraging verbal communication within the group. Each committee member, for example, can agree to pass on information to members of the group living close to them. Or personal contact can be maintained through weekly or monthly collection of subscriptions, making sure that enough time is left for a chat, which can be as important as the money.

Inevitably, groups will lose members, through waning of interest, other commitments or because they move from the area. Sometimes this process can occur with alarming rapidity. There are few things which underline more obviously the difficulties of keeping a committee together and encouraging it to remain active.

The natural process of loss of members, which contrasts with membership which declines because of misunderstanding or poor communication, will often give an edge to a group's desire to recruit new members. It is vital that a group has a continuing interest in this task, and it is as well for it to give one or more people the responsibility for ensuring the encouragement of new members. A group which has formed and is active can easily give the impression to outsiders of being exclusive, of not being interested in having new faces around. Such a situation not only runs counter to the search in neighbourhood work for openness and avoidance of cliques and elitism but is also counter-productive to the group's long-term effectiveness.

Constitutions

Community groups usually benefit from having a written constitution. This simple statement leaves open the question of when a group should adopt a constitution. It is a question which is closely linked to the formal/informal organisation debate. Without a constitution a group lacks a tangible base point which says to the rest of the world: this group exists and therefore, on the face of things, has a claim on the attention of others, as well as on other kinds of resources. Indeed, it is essential for groups to possess a constitution if they are to register with the Charity Commission, do fund-raising or if they wish to obtain council tax relief. Without a constitution, a group lays itself open to accusations of being a figment of activists' imaginations, or to expressions of scorn and dismissal as irrelevant. It is foolish for a group to risk such attacks. A constitution can be viewed in these terms as a minimal organisational requirement.

In addition, the existence of a constitution can provide a strong backbone for the internal functioning of community groups.

Not only is it there as a safety net if crises over leadership or policy arise, but it also legitimises the operating procedures of groups. These may develop intuitively with the formation of a group. The existence of a constitution will sanction them. In this way there is less likelihood of a group collapsing through confusion or disagreement over decision-making, the holding of elections or the accountability of committees or subparts of a group. Most medium-sized and large organisations will need to work a lot with a committee system. It is essential for the remit, responsibility and accountability of any committee to be clear, and the existence of a constitution can at least provide an agreed basis for reaching clarity.

Once again, different kinds of groups will require different constitutions. Some, like playgroups, community associations and citizens advice bureaux, meet few problems as they can draw upon model constitutions devised by their national bodies. Many tenants' associations in cities make use of the constitution drawn up by a federation of associations. Often, however, a suitable constitution will not be available for community groups, and a group will have to spend time on amending a constitution to meet its own requirements.

Constitutions and rules should be seen as enabling devices. Groups should use them as guidelines, not feel enslaved by them. Discussing constitutional issues can be helpful in working out and agreeing what a group is for.

Premises

The availability or otherwise of a meeting place can have a profound effect on a community group as it struggles to become a strong organisation. We stress availability and access as opposed to ownership or tenancy. The latter raise different problems which we touch upon in Chapter 10. Our concern here is to draw attention to the need for a group to have some certainty about where it can meet. This can apply at both operational and psychological levels.

It is a waste of a group's time and energy for it always to have to check out and negotiate the use of a room or building whenever it wants to meet. There will be many other things claiming the attention of organisers at this point, and they should not have to worry about a venue for meeting as well. There is good sense in clearing away this particular hurdle at one go. Thus, if the group is a small one, agreement could be reached that meetings should rotate round each member's home (in such a case, it is wise to warn against a process of competing hospitality as the group moves round; tea and biscuits one week can become sandwiches and cake the next, and can lead to unnecessary and distracting unease within the group!). For other groups, there is a need to establish a presence in particular premises – a tenants' hall, a local school, a church hall or community centre – so that there is a high expectation that it can use them again as it wants and not have to hunt around for alternatives.

Sometimes there will be overlap between premises used by a neighbourhood worker or community project, that is, as an office base, and the meeting place of a group. The combination of both in one set of premises would seem to offer potential benefits to both parties – workers and local groups. For example, a community care project in Kincardine, Fife, which was seeking to use a community development approach, found the combination invaluable:

> The local office was used as a work base and contact point for people in the community. A community newsletter and information board help groups and individuals to contact one another. From being a council facility, the office came to be more of a community focus.
>
> (Barr *et al.*, 2001: 15)

Yet ease of access to workers can place heavy pressures on them – it can be too easy for a group to turn to the worker to carry out activities which should be undertaken by the group, or the worker may come to be seen by the group as belonging only to it, whereas in reality the worker may be supporting several groups in the area. A variation on shared premises is for premises used initially by a worker or project to become, at a later stage, a resource for the community. This can happen when workers are on a short-term contract – on completion of a worker's tasks, a group can start using the premises in which he or she had been based.

A community group's need for premises will often change as it changes. Here, we have suggested that availability of a regular and agreed location can contribute to the early organisational development of groups.

Degrees of formality

The question of degree of formality of a community group can pose a dilemma:

> On the one hand, informality is essential to permit expressive relationships to develop and for members to find satisfaction in the group. Conversely, however, if groups are to develop into institutional-relations organisations, rules have to be explicated, roles specified and other formal mechanisms evolved.
>
> (Brager and Specht, 1973)

The neighbourhood worker has to help groups attain a balance between the need for informality and the development of formal structure. There will always be varieties of structures for groups of the same type, and the worker needs to remain aware of this when she or he makes suggestions to groups about how to organise. Increasingly, workers become aware of the need for groups to formalise themselves sooner rather than later. This is because of the widespread existence of partnership boards and the importance of groups being represented on them. It is difficult to do this without a group being properly constituted.

In striving to get the balance right for groups, the worker may be guided by the following considerations:

1 *How a group comes together* may help determine its structure. The group that forms around local informal networks should not ignore them when it decides upon its structure.
2 Analysis of *the function of a group* can help to determine structure. Thus a single issue or specialised group, like a playgroup, may be able to continue with a relatively informal structure compared with an organisation which seeks to speak for all the people in an area.
3 Members of a group will need *varying lengths of time* to respond to proposals for organising and the worker should be alert to indications that the group is moving too quickly for some members.
4 It can be helpful for a worker to *estimate the pros and cons of proposed types of organisation* as openly as possible with a group. How far he or she can do this will depend on the worker's relationship with a group and whether there are members who hold strong views on structure. These are often brought from other situations, such as the workplace or politics. How a group will be structured should reflect who the people are and how used they are to getting together.

5   When a group decides to adopt more formal procedures, or conversely when it opts for an informal structure having used a formal one, *changes will occur in the group*. The worker needs to be aware of these and act if necessary. Thus a sensitive area, in the shift of a group from informal to formal organisation, will be that of leadership, because the power and influence of a chairperson or secretary will become more explicit to members. Competition for leadership may accordingly increase. At the same time a worker can notice that a group which has been very anxious to establish formal procedures will often, once they have been obtained, neglect some of them and begin creating informal procedures. It is not, therefore, as if the move from informal to formal is a once-for-all matter. Rather it can be viewed as a continuum along which groups move unpredictably.

6   Neighbourhood workers need to be aware of how *new approaches to organising in a related field or movement* can be of direct relevance to their work. A significant example has been the women's movement and the innovatory ideas for organising that developed from it. The very fluid, social media-based groupings that are emerging are likely to become more accepted as a model, albeit they are not organisations in a conventional sense. Workers can never afford to remain blinkered to developments which can inform their own approaches to helping groups establish appropriate organisational arrangements. Some groups, for example, have decided to let everyone who wants to, have a turn at chairing meetings and then make a decision about whether a permanent chairperson should be elected.

7   Finally, *the position of minority or oppressed group members* should be considered. In some communities, women remain reluctant to take on a chairing role, or are intimidated by formality. Members of minority ethnic groups, people with physical disabilities and other minorities can often feel themselves to be trapped in a marginalised position. It is essential for the worker to address this situation, providing strong support for minorities and challenging assumptions and discrimination by other members of the community (and beyond).

Tactics and strategies

Increased confidence in the purpose of a community group, and a growth in commitment to it by its members, should be at the front of a neighbourhood worker's mind in building an organisation. Relevant organisational structure is necessary for any group. It is by no means sufficient. Indeed, on its own it will be arid. The essential accompaniment is the acquisition of organising experience by a group. Only with this kind of experience will people appreciate the extent of their shared need, opportunity or problem. It can take the form, on the one hand, of assigning roles and tasks to different members of a group. In this way, jobs which include the production of posters, using the Internet, distribution of a newsletter and establishing links with local newspapers together form part of a process whereby a strong group identity is created.

The other form of organising experience builds on the idea of collective activity, in contrast to the tasks referred to earlier, which can seem more individualistic even though they are being undertaken on behalf of a group. A worker's encouragement of a group to act with a collective purpose should focus on two areas: the strategic and the tactical.

Strategy is concerned with the long-term, and it implies consciously planned action based, as far as possible, on an understanding of cause and effect of a particular state of affairs. It assumes a rudimentary analysis of power and it presupposes political knowledge of the influence, strengths and weaknesses of relevant individuals and organisations.

Tactics are best conceived as methods of action, using resources to attain goals or objectives. They are to do with anticipating the moves of others, and with the consequent detailed planning and manoeuvring.

A range of tactics does not add up to a strategy. Tactics are the equivalent of a planned series of battles, not a war. A war presupposes broad, underpinning strategies on the part of contestants. Yet tactics are more than skirmishes. They should be considered moves which relate to each other in a loose logical way. A community project may adopt a strategy of working towards better local understanding of the housing market; the tactics it deploys could include research into local authority and housing association allocation policies, supporting housing groups and analysing tenure patterns.

A community group may aim to achieve better housing and recreational facilities in an area by securing increased participation of local people in decision-making processes which affect the area. This can be classed as a strategy. It will engage, however, in successive clusters of tactical actions. It will also, if it is wise, set less ambitious targets and achieve them before setting new ones. Finally, it will prepare itself on a number of fronts: collection of information, formulation of arguments, finding out where best to present arguments and how, establishment of an internal system for keeping copies of correspondence, emails and so on.

All these activities will demonstrate that a group is thinking in tactical as well as strategic terms. Alongside them, specific pieces of action will occur: organising a petition, leafleting an area, a demonstration, fund-raising events. By themselves, each one of these actions would have minimal impact. They need to be seen by members of the group concerned to relate to each other, to contain their own dynamic movement towards a particular target or set of objectives.

Introducing the distinction between strategy and tactics at this point in our discussion of the formation and building of community groups is done for two reasons. Firstly, there is a tendency for groups to organise on a 'crisis' basis. They respond to given situations – pressures, threats and opportunities. After a time, if they have not begun to form clear ideas about what they want to do and how they should do it, this becomes a very weakening and demoralising position. That theme in neighbourhood work which encourages open participation, flexible, non-bureaucratic structures and spontaneity, needs to be counterbalanced by working with groups on the need for thinking at both strategic and tactical levels. Otherwise groups will never be in control of a situation. They will always be reacting to events rather than initiating them. Countering such a tendency implies putting to a group the principle that the basis of action should not be a moral one alone but should rest on a clear plan which includes agreed tactics.

The second reason for suggesting consideration of strategies and tactics at an early stage of the organising process relates to the importance of preparing a group. Groups will have to make decisions about policy and action once they are heavily involved in issues, and they can best do this as a result of being familiar in their thinking and approach with the distinction we have made. A major task of neighbourhood workers is to help groups represent their interests to other parties effectively, and to make use of opportunities when they arise. Encouraging groups to think in strategic and tactical terms from the time that they decide to become an organisation can result in long-term benefits. There is an excellent discussion of strategies and tactics in community work in the book by Brager and Specht (1973, part IV).

The work of preparing a group for the future can be helped in at least three ways. They are as follows:

Practising

A group can be encouraged to practise skills and tactics, either by rehearsing a proposed action or by agreeing to analyse and criticise the performances of group members rigorously and openly. It could decide, in other words, to put time aside in the early period to practise and learn through doing. The support and involvement of those in leadership positions and of the neighbourhood worker involved could be crucial to such an exercise. It also lends itself to the use of video.

Members could discuss a likely scenario: a first meeting with the area regeneration team, an interview with a trust to support an application for funds, door-knocking to recruit new members. They could role play these imaginary situations, watch the video recording and pick out the weaknesses; they could then do the role play a second time, and be aware of improved confidence and the application of explicit skills. This use of video is similar to the way trainers use it in workshops on neighbourhood work. It is remarkable how many obviously weak areas can be corrected by this method; the failure, for example, of someone to introduce themselves properly at a first meeting, or the domination of an encounter by a minority of those present. Practising and rehearsing in this way can be equally useful for community groups.

Clarifying the worker's role

We have emphasised already the need for workers to make their role and relationship with the groups as clear as possible. Often at the early stage of a group's formation this will be difficult, and should not be insisted upon. However, as a group gains strength, from a sense of solidarity as well as from getting itself organised, the need for workers to clarify their role, stating what they can do for the group, becomes more relevant. This can be particularly important if a worker is both an enabler and a member of a group; she is holding more than one role. A mental health group or a women's group would be good examples.

Workers can stimulate an awareness of their role by sometimes taking on almost a participant observer role with the group. Such a capacity to be detached from the group, while at the same time being trusted and needed by it, can be helpful to a group and not interpreted as undermining its collective identity.

Setting targets

Finally, a group's preparation can return to the matter of setting realistic objectives and understanding the target: it is no use continuing to harass the local authority manager without effect if the decision has to be taken by the housing committee. A careful and anticipatory discussion of what a group can hope to achieve within an approximate time period can be salutary, and result in some reformulating or modification of early objectives. This can be of lasting value.

A group is likely to survive and be effective if its members know that each of them will carry through the responsibilities they have agreed to undertake. A testing-out process, whereby expectations on individual members and the group as a whole are assessed, can be an essential part of the growth of any group's political literacy. Such a familiarity with political processes has to include how a group manages its affairs, how control is exercised, how decisions are made and how responsibilities are allocated.

Group cohesion

Neighbourhood workers tend to talk enthusiastically about their work; those who do not will generally move on. In catching and conveying the excitement of neighbourhood work, however, they may unconsciously sidestep some of the major blockages and frustrations experienced by a group once it has decided to organise. The pattern, in reality, of the development of most groups is uneven. There may be a lengthy period while a group awaits a reply from the local authority about resources or a meeting. It is in situations like these that the neighbourhood worker has to work hard to keep a group together. Although it may be intent upon achieving its organisational goals, it will remain vulnerable to unexpected buffets, changes of plan, personality conflicts or struggles for leadership.

Here we focus briefly on the tasks of workers in looking after the internal processes of a group, compared with 'external' tasks such as broadening a group's constituency and building 'outside' support or coalitions for a group. The latter tend to form a more central part of the organising process. We have referred to them earlier in this chapter and they retain a major importance throughout the neighbourhood work process – to a greater extent perhaps than the need for internal work at the organisation-building stage. The aim of any internal work undertaken with a group will be to ensure its continuing cohesion and to encourage further growth of a sense of unity and collective purpose. Some of the forms it can take are as follows:

1   *Countering depression within a group about apparent lack of progress or unanticipated obstacles.* This can be because of consistently low turn-outs at meetings organised by the group, for example, or failure to obtain an early inflow of funds for the group, or unexpected opposition from another group of local people, or simply an entrenched and demoralising feeling that whatever the group does it will have no significant effect. Somehow the worker has to find ways of trying to help a group move away from a feeling of being 'down' in this way. The worker can refer to the achievements of groups in other similar areas. She can point to evidence of a group's work which justifies hopefulness rather than despair. She can suggest new activities and introduce discussion of different tactics. Clearly, however, the worker will not be armed with instant panaceas. Often it will be a matter of helping hold a group together until it rediscovers its sense of purpose by itself. Sometimes it is best to help a group to close down.

2   *Working with leaders individually.* Every neighbourhood worker will have a preferred style of operation. Some workers, for example, will keep formal meetings

and documentation to a minimum and utilise a range of informal skills, while others will prefer the reverse. This is partly a question of individual preference or predisposition and partly a value question about how directive a worker decides to be. Most workers, however, see the need to work closely with the leadership of a group in its early days, with a lot of emphasis being placed on bolstering the confidence of leaders. This can best be done individually, and much of the time of a worker can be spent in informal discussion with a chairperson or secretary in his or her home. It represents the private, face-to-face dimension of neighbourhood work in contrast to the more familiar public nature of the work.

It is important for that kind of support not to be limited to designated leaders of a group but to include others who play leading roles – the ideas person, for example, or the practical person. The worker can help to ensure that there are more than one or two leaders in a group, and thereby prevent it from becoming dominated by a small clique. As well as providing support in this way to individual members, the worker can also share her concerns about the group. These can include the need to expand the leadership of the group, despite the problems this sometimes poses.

It is also essential to try to avoid leadership or the initial nucleus of a group from becoming skewed in favour of the higher status or socio-economic groupings within a community. There is abundant evidence to show that participation is not uniformly distributed throughout a community. If a worker thinks that a minority section or a significant part of the neighbourhood is not represented in the group, she should share her anxiety openly with the leadership. It will usually be easier, and more productive, to do this early on in the life of a group, when there may exist more flexibility and openness, rather than leave it for later.

3   *Assessing the pace of activity by a group.* A worker's frequent contact with the leaders of a group needs to be complemented by a critical view of the pace being set for the group as a whole. Is it appropriate to the aims and objectives of the group? Is it too fast or too slow for the total group, as opposed to a majority or minority within it? A worker who is part of a community development or regeneration team is at an advantage when doing this kind of assessment because she can check it with colleagues.

The worker has to be prepared to give her views to a group she is supporting, even if this may cause some irritation within the group. The worker may feel, for example, that the plans and programmes of a group are advancing too far ahead of the process of acquiring particular skills among members, and she would argue for time being spent on developing them – chairing a meeting, public speaking, keeping accounts. We continue discussion of the worker's role in furthering the development of a group in Chapter 9.

Public meetings

In Chapter 6 we discussed the public meeting as a way of initially contacting people. We return to public meetings here in order to indicate some of their other functions. Such a discussion is particularly opportune because it may correct any impression conveyed of a clear dividing line between the work of forming an organisation and that of building it. In practice the two situations run together. We have used the distinction, in the same way that a neighbourhood worker might use it when reflecting upon her practice, in order to draw attention to particular tasks and skills within the formation and building stages. Examining the topic of public meetings, which are frequently the focus of neighbourhood work, may help to draw together the themes of forming and building and to demonstrate the major characteristics of the worker's role.

The decision of a group to hold a public meeting is frequently its first major endeavour to test the interest and support of its wider constituency. Implicit in the decision will usually be a desire both to confirm the work of the organising group and to draw in more members.

In such situations, a fledgling group is investing and risking a lot in a public meeting, and it is vital that the group gets it right. The key to this may lie in the extent of a group's awareness that the public meeting is *its* meeting. This is particularly important if councillors or outsiders are invited. They must not dominate the meeting.

A public meeting needs to be seen as one part of an organising strategy and not as an isolated event, and there must be total clarity about the purpose of a meeting: is it to find out what local people feel are the key issues? Or it is to obtain approval from those present to the issues that a group has identified already? Alternatively, a public meeting might be arranged as a recruiting device – to strengthen the membership of a group – or to increase a group's profile as a result of publicity. The latter can be an important way of showing to local agencies the strength and potential of a group, especially if senior councillors and officers of the local authority are invited.

A group needs to work on the issue of 'why hold a meeting?' in relation to its other activities and plans. Then, when it moves ahead with organising the meeting, it can retain some control over it by drawing upon the strategic and tactical thinking we have suggested a group needs to engage in from the beginning. Table 7.2 illustrates some of the opportunities available to a group when it is entirely responsible for organising a meeting, and contrasts it with the situation of a group entering a meeting where it has little idea of what to expect.

Planning and management of public meetings calls for skilful judgement by a neighbourhood worker as well as by community groups. In a sense, issues around a public meeting epitomise the demands made upon two main skill areas throughout the forming and building process: an excellent sense of timing – when to introduce specific ideas and techniques to an evolving group; and an ability to think strategically and to be able to convey such an approach to community groups.

Table 7.2 Preparing for a public meeting

	Strategies	*Tactics*
Known situation	Why have it? Who should be there? What do we want from it? Who will organise what?	Leaflets and posters, newsletter and website, rehearsal, seating arrangement, prepared questions, priming the press
Unknown situation	Who will be there? What are we all agreed on? What kind of meeting is it – exchange of opinions or negotiating?	Clarify purpose, suggest seating alteration, adjournment, spokesperson, note-taker

Timing and strategy both retain their importance throughout the organising process, but they first attain major significance at this stage. Both, it should be said, sometimes appear to be handled by workers and groups intuitively or by hunch: a worker, for example, who had been involved with a small group of tenants for more than a year and who had been unable to link it with a youth group he was also working with on the same estate, decided to attend what he thought would be another inconclusive meeting. To his surprise, membership had revived, and during the meeting sufficiently positive comments were made about the value of the youth activities being organised for him to suggest that the two groups should get together in order to improve facilities on the estate. The group agreed to it. The worker could think of no rational explanation for this development. Like a lot of neighbourhood work, it was a combination of the place, the time and the people.

We are aware of the danger of implying that every group will move, with varying degrees of difficulty, through the formation and building phases. Clearly they will not. Many informal groups will fail to become organisations. Others will spring into life spontaneously, as we see in the following two examples:

1. The Grenfell Tower fire on 14th June 2017 killed 72 people. The action group which formed immediately, Grenfell United, was made up of victims' family members and survivors. It has campaigned ceaselessly not only for the local authority, Kensington and Chelsea, to accept responsibility for the fire, caused by allowing cheap cladding to be used on the outside of the building, but also for a national social housing regulator and for all dangerous materials, to be banned and removed from houses. It is a remarkable example of how community action can be effective and strategic.

2. 'The exemplary case is Rotterdam, where in response to the closure of local libraries in 2011 a group of residents created a reading room from an old Turkish bathhouse. The project began with a festival of plays, films and discussions, then became permanently embedded. It became a meeting place where people could talk, read and learn new skills – and soon began, with some help from the council, to spawn restaurants, workshops, care cooperatives, green projects, cultural hubs and craft collectives. These projects inspired other people to start their own. One estimate suggests that there are now 1,300 civic projects in the city. Deep cooperation and community-building now feels entirely normal there'.

(George Monbiot, 2017)

It is important to note that in both examples the local action spread to city-wide and national contexts.

References

Alinsky, S. (1969) *Reveille for radicals*, New York: Vintage Books.
Baldock, P. (1974) *Community work and social work*, London: Routledge & Kegan Paul.
Barr, A., Stenhouse, C. and Henderson, P. (2001) *Caring communities. A challenge for social inclusion*, York: York Publishing Services.
Brager, G. and Specht, H. (1973) *Community organising*, New York: Columbia University Press.
Cary, L. J. (1970) 'The role of the citizen in the community development process', in L. J. Cary (ed.) *Community development as a process*, Columbia: University of Missouri Press.

Chanan, G. (1997) *Active citizenship and community involvement*, Dublin: European Foundation for the Improvement of Living and Working Conditions.

Gilchrist, A. (2019) *The well-connected community: a networking approach to community development* (3rd edn), Bristol: The Policy Press.

Joseph Rowntree Foundation. (1999) 'Neighbourhood images in Teeside', in *Findings*, York: JRF.

Joseph Rowntree Foundation. (2010) 'Participation and community on Bradford's traditionally white estates', in *Findings*, York: JRF.

Monbiot, G. (2017) 'This is how we take back control: from the bottom-up', *The Guardian*, 8 February.

Sloman, A. (2012) 'Using participatory theatre in international community development', *Community Development Journal*, 47, 1: 42–57.

8 Helping to clarify goals and priorities

Clarifying goals	Issues for the worker
Identifying priorities	Role
Nominal groups	Framework for action
Delphi	Constraints on workers
	Recording
	Standing back

The need for community groups to clarify goals and identify priorities is integral to the forming and building of organisations discussed in the last chapter. They are necessarily linked to strategy formation. Clarification of goals and the identification of priorities are also closely connected with each other. Sometimes a more formal approach to this stage of the neighbourhood work process can be used. Fiona Ballantyne (personal communication) suggests organising planning days which enable groups, through facilitated sessions, to:

- analyse situations, issues and needs;
- barriers to change/improvement;
- develop a vision of their area, issue or aspirations;
- set strategic goals;
- prioritise goals;
- develop action plans.

It is important to give attention to the question of how groups consciously work through the process of deciding upon goals and priorities. It is also imperative to focus on some key implications for the neighbourhood worker when a group is organised to the point of acquiring experience and gaining confidence about what it wants to achieve. We shall explore these two themes by discussing in turn the need for community groups to examine goals and set priorities. We shall then identify some issues for workers.

We preface our contribution to this area by noting that the requirement for rational thought needs to be considered within an analysis of social exclusion and community development. How meaningful will a worker's attempt be to introduce issues of choice and decision-making, based on explicit criteria, with groups many of whose members are struggling to survive? There will, in deprived neighbourhoods, be the ability to grapple with the issues, but initially there may be a lack of familiarity with them.

DOI: 10.4324/9781003310006-8

A worker may be able to highlight similarities with group members' other activities at work and in the community, such as trade unions, sports and running a household; in these activities people regularly set goals and priorities without describing it as such.

Discussion of goals and priorities will be among the more difficult tasks for community groups. Accordingly a worker needs to approach this area with sensitivity, and be prepared to adapt plans for tackling issues of choice.

Clarifying goals

There is a tendency to reify the search for clear goals or aims. They can come to seem highly abstract. Using the distinction between goals and objectives may exacerbate the dangers, yet it is a valuable distinction and one which we adopt. Goals are the highest level of objectives. They lack specificity, they stand out as statements of value and they are not easily attainable. Objectives, on the other hand, are concerned with specifics; they suggest what action is implied and what targets should be attained – they are stepping stones to goals. They relate directly to strategies and tactics. This use of the term 'objectives' has the effect of reinforcing the abstract connotation of 'goals'.

Most organisations have multiple goals rather than a single goal, and this is as true of small, newly formed community groups as it is of established organisations. Multiple goals do not necessarily imply confusion or contradiction within an organisation. In addition, organisations' goals are not static; they shift over time. Rothman (1969) suggests that it may be useful to view an organisation's goals from an historical perspective. Either one goal is substituted for another ('goal displacement') or new goals are added when old ones have been achieved or cannot be obtained ('goal succession').

Goal development is an ongoing process, which is 'all the more complicated by the fact that there are three actors (i.e. constituents, workers and sponsors) attempting to influence the outcome'. Brager and Specht also suggest three ways in which organisations can deal with differences among goals:

> (1) When the objectives are viewed by participants as compatible, compromise is possible, and two goals may be sought at once; (2) a second form of compromise is accomplished by 'planned ambiguity', a form of adjustment which occurs when a group's objectives seem to conflict; (3) the third method is to achieve clarity by choosing one goal as primary from among conflicting claims, discarding others, or assigning them a lower priority.
>
> (Brager and Specht, 1973)

The example they provide for the first form of compromise, the welfare rights movement, is as appropriate to the UK context as to the United States: those in leadership positions frequently see the mobilisation of claimants as a means of bringing about change in the benefits system, but claimants are often intent on achieving more modest and short-range ends, such as an increase in the number of grants and loans available. There is evidence to suggest the feasibility of retaining both goals at the same time. However, the difficulties of doing so should not be underestimated.

The idea of planned ambiguity of goals is given considerable significance by Brager and Specht because ambiguity is 'more advantageous to the *least* powerful members of the coalition': the clearer the goals, the more influential become existing leaders of a group or organisation, 'in effect, the precise goals of organisations represent the clarity of their most powerful members'. The advantages of planned goal ambiguity will clearly make considerable demands on the worker's skills.

Within community work literature, Rothman (1969) has shown how specific objectives are inherent in community work practice, but they exist alongside less tangible 'process goals'. The latter refer – in simple terms – to educational aims, whereby local people, through their experience of organising together, develop and change as individuals and groups. They are broad goals which are focused on 'growth' or 'maturity' in civic affairs rather than on the solution of a particular problem or the meeting of a special need. We have seen how it is associated in particular with the work of Ross, the Biddles and Batten. It has been taken up by both those concerned to evolve new forms of adult education and the followers of 'consciousness-raising' methods articulated by Freire. It contrasts with the achievement by community groups of specific tasks. Rothman suggests that the use of the terms 'process' and 'task' goals causes confusion, partly because process goals often contain concrete tasks. Our purpose here is not to pursue this argument but to emphasise the tension which often faces a community group between sustaining its own cohesion and fixing on a clear set of goals and objectives.

In what ways can there exist tension or competing claims between the internal functioning of a community group and the clarification of goals and objectives? In earlier chapters we have referred to the importance of a group developing a collective identity, and how this can often begin through social relationships and informal interchanges which help to bind people to a group. As a group turns towards working out in specific terms what it intends to achieve, the 'togetherness' and unity of the group may be put under strain. Basically this happens because differences of view about the group's goals emerge. There are at least four ways in which this can happen.

1   *Pressures on members*. Strong personal disagreements may be exposed, which often are inseparable from conflicts of personalities. This can occur once the effects of a group's activities begin to be recognised in the community or by agencies, and the group thereby experiences both positive and negative pressures. The message is driven home that being a member of a group can have serious implications for the individual. It is one thing, for example, when a group announces it is to become a member of a regeneration partnership, but those involved will face a quite different kind of reality when they experience the pressures of attending meetings and seek to provide feedback to a wider constituency. It is then that those most committed to the group's partnership role will be perceived by other members as 'the most powerful individuals'. They will, accordingly, be able to place their stamp on the group's functioning, because they become the leaders in a situation of covert disagreement among the membership or constituency about the group's goals.

2   *Formal and informal priorities*. It is quite possible for a group to retain its 'celebratory' element, the socialising, the fun and enjoyment which form such a vital part of neighbourhood work, with the furthering of more serious activities. Indeed, both a neighbourhood worker and a group's leaders will usually strive to ensure that these do not become lost as the group increases its 'work' activity. There is always a close connection between the informal and the formal elements of neighbourhood work.

Inevitably, however, some members will feel less committed to furthering a group's main aims than others. The important point for the group is not to allow that natural division or sets of preferences to divide it. Those people who are seen to do the 'small tasks' – social secretary, delivering envelopes, locking up – or who cannot give as much time to the group's work as others, need to receive recognition of their contributions by those who set the pace of the group in terms of its main work. Otherwise the group will lose them, and be so much the weaker.

3   *Conflicts of interest.* There will often be clear-cut conflicts of interest within a group which are only revealed as its goals become clarified. Such conflict may turn upon differences of viewpoint, values, ideology between individuals about proposed policies and actions, or it may emerge as the issue or content area with which the group is concerned is better understood. An example might be a local authority's development plan for an area; if an individual is only going to be minimally affected by it, he or she is less likely to stay an active member of a group campaigning to stop it. In neighbourhood work it is essential for a worker and a group to be able to judge when certain goals have or have not been achieved. In the latter case, if conflicts of interest become counter-productive or 'planned ambiguity' loses its validity, it may become necessary for a worker to help a group to stop meeting.

4   *Ends and means.* It is artificial to study goals without relating them to the means or methods by which they are to be attained, or without recognising that the two interact. How you are going to achieve something can be as important for some people, in terms of their involvement, as what it is proposed to achieve. Some people, for example, will support a housing association which aims to extend housing availability but will relinquish that support if the association decides to support the setting up of housing cooperatives. In that case there can be no disagreement about goals, but divergence about how to achieve them. We shall see in Chapter 10 how there can be fundamental differences between a group's decision to provide a service and a decision to campaign, and how they may each rely upon different individuals to support them.

Management specialists have developed a number of formats and step-by-step guidelines for goal and objectives setting. These can be used to ensure that actions both derive from and contribute to social and individual values. One approach which may be of particular use to neighbourhood workers is that called the 'key results' exercise, because it can be undertaken by individuals and small groups. It is essentially a method of relating the targets and objectives of the individual to the goals of an organisation to enable the one to help determine the other. It allows individuals and small groups to be clearer in their work, to have a strong measure of self-control, to make explicit their activities and to be self-regulating and self-appraising.

The 'key results' exercise is set out in the following as a very simple planning schema. It should be changed around to suit the particular circumstances of groups.

- *Goals/objectives.* What overall improvements do you personally want to see achieved in the next year? Make sure that you are talking about effects to be achieved rather than activities.
- *Evaluative criteria.* How will you know you have achieved any of the goals or objectives – marginally, substantially or completely?

- *Action*. What activities do you need to undertake to achieve your goals/objectives?
- *Blockages*. Who or what will prevent your achievement of goals/objectives? What will you do to counteract these blockages?

Neighbourhood workers may find the material emanating from management literature and training too restrictive or find its terminology off-putting. The material, however, can be useful for groups. It can also help a worker's planning. The book on capacity building by Skinner (2006) is relevant because it locates techniques and skills, many of which originate from management studies, within a community development framework. The book by Miller (2008) sets out key issues about managing community development. The handbook by Nick Wates remains a useful resource for helping groups plan. It contains suggestions on how planning days can be organised and which methods can be used (Wates, 2000).

Before we discuss the question of the identification of a group's priorities, it is important to emphasise the crucial part that goal clarification plays in the neighbourhood work process. It is, first, an essential link between a worker finding out about a neighbourhood and the development of a strategy and programme which will be relevant to that neighbourhood. The groups he or she comes to work with need to be aware of that connection. Their growth cannot be divorced from the actions and thinking of the worker.

Failure to think through the goals of a group is frequently the weakest point in a group's life and in the organising process. It is when confusion, frustration or failure is most likely to happen. Once again, we see the need for choices about a group's direction to be strategic ones. An approach should be selected with a view to achieving specified goals and objectives, not just in order to make a statement. Furthermore, strategy about goals can reach out well beyond the neighbourhood where a group is active.

Second, spending time and energy on a group's goals is essential if the idea of evaluation is to retain validity. Without clarity about goals, there will be nothing against which to measure the achievements which may be claimed. As a result, the continuing sense of movement of the process idea becomes lost. It comes to be a once-and-for-all device rather than a flexible, cyclical one, and considerably less useful as a result.

Identifying priorities

The importance of a worker helping a group turn their discontent into a series of needs, the needs into a range of objectives and the objectives into tasks and priorities is of critical importance, not least because of the diversity of needs and problems that people may experience. Again and again we can see in neighbourhood work the extent to which groups have to put together a strategy which both takes account of the breadth of needs, objectives and tasks and which sets clear priorities.

Choice of priorities needs to be based upon criteria, rather than (for example) upon impulse or upon 'what seems best'. By criteria one means, in this context, agreed and articulated reasons why a group chooses to concentrate upon one issue or project rather than another; for example, a group proceeds with organising children's playschemes because it thinks children need those kinds of opportunities provided by the group, rather than because facilities for playschemes happen to be available and no other agency is planning to organise them.

Identifying and setting priorities is therefore an essential part of helping a group to plan effectively, a point underlined in a good practice guide to community development produced by the Community Foundation for Northern Ireland:

> The plan should be ambitious but realistic, so that it creates motivation, enthusiasm and, most importantly, it produces results. A group will normally make several plans of action in its lifetime so it will not be necessary to fit everything into the first two years.; it is important not to aim beyond what you know you can achieve in that time.
>
> (www.communityfoundation.org)

We have noted already that, in the process of clarifying goals, conflicts of interest are likely to emerge within a community group, and these will often be exacerbated as priorities are decided upon. A group may intend to be a multifunctional organisation from the beginning, or it may have formed in order to protest over a single issue 'and in the course of making that protest has established recreational and welfare activities for the sake of raising money and morale and that these activities now seem valuable in themselves' (Baldock, 1974). In both situations, debate about which functions or programmes to concentrate on after an initial phase of activity is likely to bring different interests and viewpoints into overt conflict with each other, and oblige the group to live through a crisis. This is a particularly important issue when community groups are being encouraged to become social enterprises: the balance between financial viability and meeting social outcomes becomes critical. Baldock also points out that:

> Where a distinct shift in priorities appears to be required, then this may imply a change of leadership. The leadership thrown up on the first instance may be of people committed purely to one view of what the association should do or with talents that are most appropriate to the initial phase, such as charismatic individuals. It is not uncommon for groups at this stage of development to enter into overt conflict situations in which the early leaders are ejected from their position or alternatively for a group to fail to change its leadership and begin to stagnate.
>
> (Baldock, 1974)

Changing direction and the turnover of leadership can be considered a normal occurrence in neighbourhood work. Similarly, we should expect the priorities of both multifunctional and single-issue organisations to change.

While it is easy to explain the need for groups to identify priorities, to make choices as to what they will do, it is much harder to provide guidelines or models of *how* priorities can be identified. Very often discussing the issues in group meetings can be unrewarding. It can lead to increased ill feeling among group members, and the group can fail to arrive at agreed decisions. For a group to experience such failure at a critical stage in its development can be disastrous, and every attempt should be made to prevent it.

We are aware that the nature of neighbourhood work implies a high degree of unpredictability; things happen as a result of a wide range of factors – from how local service agencies are perceived by residents, to the intuitions of activists and workers. Nevertheless, there do exist models and techniques developed in other disciplines, which can be adapted and used to help community groups reach decisions and make choices about action and programmes. These are worth examining by neighbourhood workers and community groups – even if they subsequently decide to reject them – in order to tighten up on this crucial but weak area of organising. Two techniques of which we have had experience are the *nominal group technique* and the *Delphi technique*. We propose to summarise these here but we advise workers who plan to use them to (a) study the original source material, (b) consider how they might adapt the material to their particular situations and (c) look at other techniques, for example, story dialogue, open space, world café method and appreciative enquiry.

Nominal groups

The nominal group technique, developed from social psychology studies of Delbecq and Van de Ven, offers:

> A planning sequence which seeks to provide an orderly process of structuring the decision-making of groups, fragmented in terms of vested interests, rhetorical and ideological concepts, and differentiated expertise, needed to be brought together in order for a programme to emerge or change to take place.
>
> (Delbecq and Van de Ven, 1971)

This suggests its possible appropriateness for community groups facing the kinds of choices we are discussing. It is a group process model for situations where there exists uncertainty or possible disagreement about choices, and it can be used for (a) identifying strategic problems and (b) developing appropriate and innovative programmes to solve them. It originated from studies of decision meetings and programme planning in a community action agency during the United States' War on Poverty i n the 1960s.

The model contains five phases, and for each phase there are specific group techniques and specific roles for different interest groups. The phases are problem exploration, knowledge exploration, priority development, programme development and programme evaluation. One of the objectives is to facilitate innovation and creativity in planning. Its reliance upon nominal groups (groups in which individuals work in the presence of one another but remain silent) builds upon research studies which indicate the superiority of such groups compared with conventional 'brainstorming' and discussion groups.

Two other important features of the technique are, first, the separation of 'personal' from organisational' problems: a large meeting is divided into groups of six to nine people, and each individual is asked to write 'personal feelings' on one side of a card and 'organisational difficulties' on the other side. The person managing the exercise then asks all members of the groups to spend 30 minutes listing aspects of the problem on their cards without speaking to anyone. He or she then asks one person from each group to record on a common sheet written comments of the members of each group. The groups are then given 30 minutes to review their lists – they can clarify, elaborate or defend any item, or add items. Each member is then asked privately to vote on the five items he or she considers most crucial on the 'personal' problem list: this represents the end of the first phase of the technique. The remaining four phases require a similar form of structuring.

A second notable feature of the technique is the use of the round-robin procedure, which allows each group member to offer an idea; as a result, less secure members will feel more able to follow the risk-taking of more secure members.

The nominal group process provides both quantitative data in the sense of voted-upon priorities and qualitative data in terms of a rich, descriptive discussion which follows the nominal group activity, in which members often provide critical incidents or personal anecdotes.

While the technique seems to relate more obviously to professional groupings, its methods are also very relevant to community groups, and use has been made of them by neighbourhood workers. It deliberately and systematically structures the business of deciding upon priorities. The point to stress is the need to adapt and modify the technique as developed by Delbecq and Van de Ven to suit both a neighbourhood work context and specific situations. We would certainly not advise uncritical transfer of the technique from the social planning context described by the authors to a neighbourhood work setting.

The nominal group technique is one of the main methods used in the running of Future Workshops, an educational technique which has been adapted for widespread use by neighbourhood work, planning and group work trainers.

Delphi

We also advise adaptation to those who decide to make use of the Delphi technique. This aims to develop scenarios based on expert knowledge of related topics.

The technique is no more than a device which can be used when the agreement of 'experts' on an uncertain issue is desired. Although it originated in forecasting and futurist opinion gathering, it has also been used in industrial decision-making, educational planning and studies in the quality of life. It is claimed to be a rapid and relatively efficient way to 'cream the tops of the heads' of a group of knowledgeable people.

Its three main features are anonymity, controlled feedback and statistical group response. It focuses primarily on identifying items of dissatisfaction among participants:

> In using the method, anonymity is effected through questionnaires or other formal communication devices. This reduces the effect on the group that might be produced by dominant individuals. Controlled feedback is used to reduce noise usually encountered in face-to-face conferences. The exercise is conducted as a sequence of rounds in which the results of the previous rounds are fed back to the participants. The statistical group response is a device to assure that the opinion of every member of the group is represented in the final response.
>
> (Molnar and Kammerud, 1975)

Although the highly structured nature of the Delphi technique and its emphasis on the role of the expert may appear alien to the style and values of community work, it would be short-sighted for workers to dismiss it and other similar techniques out of hand. Most of them have been tested and shown to produce measurable benefits, particularly in situations where a large number of people have to work on complex and ill-defined problems. Local people are knowledgeable about their community, and it is axiomatic that their expertise should be used in the process of reaching decisions about what issues to work on. The Delphi method is simple in concept and there is a great deal of latitude in the specifics of carrying it out.

Planning for Real, a planning and training method familiar to many groups and workers, normally makes use of priority charts. These allow for prioritisation into three categories of urgency: 'now', 'soon' and 'later'. They can be simply and visually displayed. Prioritising can take place during the main Planning for Real event and/or could be set up as a sequel, with different groups forming to work out the priorities on a range of issues (www.communityplanning.net). Material in a publication giving a number of techniques (New Economics Foundation, 1998) is directly relevant to priority setting; and *Equalities and communities* (Gilchrist, 2007) provides a framework for tackling inequalities within which it is important to set clear goals and measure progress against them.

Issues for the worker

At its more exhilarating and turbulent moments, the unfolding of a piece of neighbourhood work can appear to be self-evident. The cry from the heart of the worker that his job is to 'get out there and organise' is persuasive, and at such moments advice or training guides about the need to clarify roles can seem both dampening and restrictive, as well as contrary to the natural instinct of a worker.

Yet, how often has inadequate reflection upon role at different phases in a group's existence contributed to confusion or conflict both for the worker and the group? Too frequently, in our experience. The need for consideration to be given both to conceptualisation about worker issues and to specific action is, we believe, particularly pressing when, as it were, a group is 'coming of age': it has set itself in a particular direction, it knows what it seeks to achieve. It has gone past the earlier phase of forming itself into a group, and it is not yet faced with problems of maintaining itself or providing services. This 'growth' period of a group should prompt a worker to re-examine his own contribution and tasks.

Role

In Chapter 5 we use the term 'role predisposition', because we think a worker's decision about role should be determined partially by the situations in which he and a group find themselves. In that a group has acquired evident strength and sense of purpose, it will often be appropriate for the worker who has given it considerable support to begin to adopt a lower profile, to *appear* to be less intensely involved with the group. The worker will stop doing so much for the group. He will also seek to establish other ways in which to help the group in the future. It may be, for example, that a group has decided to explore the option of setting up a social enterprise and the worker may have limited experience or knowledge in that area. The worker's strength may lie more in being able to offer educational expertise. He should feel able to discuss such a situation openly with the group, and indicate the kind of support he can best offer in the future. The worker cannot be a jack-of-all-trades, and is also likely to have other work to do.

Framework for action

The effectiveness of a worker or a project will be undermined if insufficient work has been put into establishing how the worker will relate to a group once it becomes active. The use of the term 'establishing a contract' is not always appropriate in a neighbourhood work setting, whether it is used in a 'strong' or 'weak' sense, and we prefer to think of a process of open discussion or negotiation as the means by which a future working relationship is agreed upon. Neighbourhood work has, in our view, to remain a fluid and flexible activity.

However, there are situations in which agreeing a contract between a worker and a group is advisable. For example, in the 'focused, indirect' model of rural community work put forward by Francis and Henderson, this way of working is recommended because of the limited amount of contact there will be between a worker and the local people. The contract:

> Has to establish what kind of support the worker will offer, over what period of time, and with what probable outcomes. The contract will need to convey the level of flexibility which will be possible, as well as the time-scale for this level of work.
>
> (Francis and Henderson, 1992: 83)

Other situations where establishing a contract can be important are when (a) there are tensions or conflicts in a community and (b) a regeneration programme is scheduled to inject a high level of resources into a neighbourhood. In both instances, it will be particularly important for local people to know the extent of worker support on which they can rely. This was the thinking behind the contracts unit of Nottingham Community Project in the early 1980s. The senior community worker recalls:

> Instead of going into an area and saying, 'right, we're here for two years like it or leave it', you would draw up a contract with an existing community group and they would say what they wanted from you and you would negotiate with them as to what you would provide in terms of hours, the kind of input they needed, what training they wanted and you would write it up as a binding contract, renewable after six months if both sides still wanted to.
>
> (Pitchford, 2008: 83)

Our hesitation about contracts is that they risk injecting an element of artificiality and rigidity into natural human relationships. On the whole, people who are active in their neighbourhood do not want to be pinned down in terms of their precise personal commitments. Community participation should not be like that. A worker should never be in the position of appearing to control the rate of activity of a group or the ups and downs of its existence.

Whatever method a worker and a group feel most comfortable with, our chief concern is to stress the importance for the worker and the group of deciding what kind of support the worker will provide, how frequent it will be, and on what issues or areas of interest it will concentrate. We discuss what these can be in the next chapter.

Naturally, workers will continue to 'care' for the group, and do things for it, outside any formulated agreement, and fulfilling such a role can continue to be very time-consuming. Groups will continue to face internal crises of one kind or another, and a worker will either be asked to help or will feel he needs to offer guidance or support if the group is to survive. It is not easy to divide up a worker's relationship with a group, and in advocating the advantages of setting out a framework of action between worker and group we do not wish to deny the need at times for both parties to go outside it.

Constraints on workers

If a worker is faced with clear constraints in his job, then it is wise to explore with the group what these imply. Workers' discussions within their agency about what they intend to do will be tested as the pressures of work increase. Furthermore, a community group's understanding of a worker's action in moments of crisis of the group with other organisations will be helped if he has raised the general question with the group earlier. Our concern here is not to debate the question of to whom a worker owes loyalty and accountability but to suggest that it constitutes an item for discussion between a worker and a group at this stage.

Recording

Neighbourhood workers need to decide upon a manageable and relevant form of recording from the moment that they begin a community project; Baldock (1974) has pointed out that many workers write up a neighbourhood analysis, based on their impressions and recordings, after about six months, and recording the progress of a group's formation is vital. However, writers who have discussed recording in neighbourhood work draw attention to the need for a worker to adopt a well-organised recording system once he is working with a group on a continuing basis. It is good practice for workers to be disciplined as to the amount of recording they do. In his research into the practice of community workers in Strathclyde, Barr found that a typical worker would have spent approximately two-and-a-half hours writing and one hour and 20 minutes in reading and information collection per week:

> Given the significance attached in the practice theory literature of community work to recording, monitoring and evaluation of work and the demands on workers to keep abreast of developments in their area of work, this does not appear to be a very substantial amount of time.
>
> (Barr, 1996: 33)

Baldock lists four questions a worker should have in mind when doing process recording of a group, that is, observing and noting, for example, the interactions of a group meeting:

- Did the group session achieve its purpose?
- What was the feeling of the meeting like?
- What were the different roles of individuals?
- What was the worker's role?

In deciding what kind of recording to do, it can be helpful for the worker to ensure that he does not rely on one method only. The most usual approach is to do narrative recording, on a day-to-day basis, and to mix this with recording under specific headings. If a worker is part of a team, or collaborates closely with practitioners in neighbouring areas, it is possible to agree what the headings should be and what data should be included under them. This offers an opportunity for comparative studies.

Usually, too, a worker will want to undertake his own recording, to be used essentially to help improve the worker's practice and to provide a basis for evaluation, and a more limited recording for his agency. Whatever kind of recording workers do, they will need to respect the feelings of the group with whom they are working: they should keep detailed recording of the group confidential, and they should only release information about the group for storing in the agency's records with the agreement of the group.

Once again, the need for workers to talk this and other worker-related issues through with the group is underlined. So, too, is the way in which workers' skills relate to each part of the neighbourhood process – they are in use at different times and with varying emphases. Here we have tried to show how recording by a worker can help a group to set priorities.

Standing back

We conclude by encouraging workers to keep a close watch on the tempo and ideals of a group. They may well have to urge a group to step aside from its involvement in action in order to reflect upon where it is going, to stand back occasionally and consider what members' activity means in relation to the group's goals. At the same time they may need to remind a group of what it can hope to achieve, to share with it their imagination of an improved state of affairs. Neighbourhood workers need to have a visionary and optimistic quality, and it can be useful for them to share this enthusiasm with a group as it struggles to make impact on a local or wider context. A useful framework for workers to use to aid reflection is contained in the book by Wilson and Wilde (2001: 112). A community development project which sets out an approach which combines encouraging groups to have both vision and strong organisation is the Dublin-based Community Action Network (CAN):

Typically, an organisation can be described as having four dimensions:

- Its primary purpose, vision or mission, and why it exists
- Its actions in the world, and what it does to implement its purpose
- Its organisation or how it structures itself to carry out its role
- Its relationships both internal and external: how it maintains the harmony necessary to function and how it develops the alliances it needs to succeed

We invite organisations to develop coherence across these four dimensions. For an individual organisation, this might mean revisiting or changing its primary purpose, questioning or celebrating the effectiveness of its activities, reorganising itself or attending to its internal or external relationships. This is the breadth of organisational development work.

However, there is also a depth to organisational development work. CAN believes that a healthy organisation requires more than strategic plans and management systems to be transformative and make a difference. The intangible qualities or spirit that characterises an organisation also requires attention. Our work with organisations facilitates them in becoming learning organisations (www.canaction.ie).

In itemising the aforementioned issues, which relate to this stage of the neighbourhood work process, we have made a somewhat artificial distinction between the launching of an autonomous group and its subsequent continuation. This reflects our concern to 'sharpen up' the identification of specific skill areas for different phases of neighbourhood work. In the next chapter we explore the roles and tasks of the worker when maintaining a community group, and many of these will complement the points we have discussed in this chapter.

References

Baldock, P. (1974) *Community work and social work*, London: Routledge & Kegan Paul.

Barr, A. (1996) *Practising community development. Experience in Strathclyde*, London: CDF Publications.

Brager, G. and Specht, H. (1973) *Community organising*, New York: Columbia University Press.

Delbecq, A. L. and Van de Ven, A. H. (1971) 'A group process model for problem identification and program planning', *Journal of Applied Behavioural Science* (September); also in N. Gilbert and H. Specht (eds) (1977) *Planning for welfare*, Englewood Cliffs, NJ: Prentice-Hall.

Francis, D. and Henderson, P. (1992) *Working with rural communities*, Basingstoke: Macmillan.

Gilchrist, A. (2007) *Equalities and communities: challenge, choice and change*, London: CDF.

Miller, C. (2008) *The community development challenge: management. Towards high standards in community development*, London: CDF.

Molnar, D. and Kammerud, M. (1975) 'Problem analysis: the Delphi technique', *Socio-Economic Planning Science*, 9; also in N. Gilbert and H. Specht (eds) (1977) *Planning for social welfare*, Englewood Cliffs, NJ: Prentice-Hall.

New Economics Foundation. (1998) *Participation works!* London: NEF.

Pitchford, M. with Henderson, P. (2008) *Making spaces for community development*, London: CDF.

Rothman, J. (1969) 'An analysis of goals and roles in community organisation practice', in R. Kramer and H. Specht (eds), *Readings in community organisation practice* (1st edn), Englewood Cliffs, NJ: Prentice-Hall.

Skinner, S. (2006) *Strengthening communities. A guide to capacity building for communities and the public sector*, London: CDF.

Wates, N. (2000) *The community planning handbook*, London: Earthscan.

Wilson, M. and Wilde, P. (2001) *Building practitioner strengths*, London: CDF.

9   Keeping the organisation going

Providing resources and information	Developing confidence and competence
Providing resources	Technical tasks
Providing information	Interactional tasks
Being supportive	Equal opportunities
Coordinating help	
Planning	
Policy planning	
Operations planning	

> The challenge of running the community house project is that everyone who carries out tasks does so as a volunteer, on top of their day-to-day tasks, in their spare time the extent of which is constantly changing. Therefore flexibility and internal communication are important to allow for the replacement of team members who drop out or withdraw for a period of time, to take over their tasks and to keep things rolling. Facebook, Google mailing lists and friendships within the team are essential tools to keep work organisation and communication flowing smoothly. Thanks to these, we all have closer or looser ties with team members, allowing us to know when they need help with their private lives – and we try to help each other as much as we can; at other times we see when someone has spare capacity and can take on additional tasks and responsibilities, making our work go more smoothly.
>
> (Anna Borbala Hernadi, personal communication)

These comments were made by a community worker in a rural part of Hungary. They indicate some of the issues surrounding this stage of the neighbourhood work process.

Many workers learn the hard way that community groups can be fragile. The seemingly confident group that launched itself with a blaze of publicity may plod on ineffectually, its meetings becoming more and more ritualised. Community action and community-based regeneration are often long processes. Achievements are rarely immediate. Consequently, a group becomes at risk as interests decline, personal disputes and needs intrude, and the lack of progress demoralises. Slowness and indifference in the response of a local authority or partnership board to letters from a newly formed group can sometimes be enough to ensure its withering away.

The maintenance and strengthening of the community group must be of essential interest to the worker and, indeed, to the members and officers of the group. We write 'interest' because there will be some groups who will flourish without anyone 'doing anything' about their development; on the other hand, there are many groups who may fall into dire straits if the worker has not been working hard with members to help

DOI: 10.4324/9781003310006-9

the group stay intact and develop. The strength of the group, and the confidence and competence of its members are thus legitimate matters of concern for the neighbourhood worker, whose contribution to group management has been described by Barr:

> In deprived areas residents experience many pressures and internal divisions within the community which may be reflected in the way that group members behave towards one another. Indeed, some groups may be so torn by internal divisions that they are never able to represent effectively the interests of their area. Given that this is so, the enabling process within community work is centrally concerned with holding the disparate elements of groups together, and encouraging the group to adopt a collective view of its goals and methods which reflect the needs and views of the area as a whole. This role is often extremely time- consuming and exacting but is an essential prerequisite to effective work by groups. In many respects it is the skill of a community worker in this role that is most important in determining the success of the community work process, yet it is the role which is least visible to outsiders.
>
> (Barr, 1977)

Tasks such as helping a group get through a depression or crisis, or assisting individuals to learn new skills and develop in a particular office in the group, may be best approached through understanding the approach adopted by the worker, and the force of his own personality, energy and enthusiasm in motivating members. It is often the quality of the worker's relationships, and the strength of his own commitment to the group's work, that contribute most to the task of helping to maintain the organisation. If a worker has been key to the setting up of a group, he is more likely to be more involved in a group than if he has not.

It is possible to provide a number of ways of conceptualising the group maintenance tasks of the neighbourhood worker. While there is some overlap, each can contribute to a particular dimension of the task.

Group maintenance may be portrayed in terms of theories about small group behaviour: the ability to work effectively in both small and large groups, to help people organise themselves into a group and to work towards their goals. It also includes skill at understanding group processes and dynamics and helping people to present the essentials of their work and their activities.

The 'group work' perspective emphasises the dynamics of the group, as well as the phases or stages of growth through which the group might progress. Brager and Specht (1973), for example, describe group development in terms of four stages and indicate the kinds of tasks for the workers who are present at each stage.

Another slant on the tasks of group maintenance is implicit in those descriptions of the worker's role that stress facilitating, enabling, supporting and encouraging appropriate behaviour. Murray Ross (1967) describes the tasks of the enabling role as:

- focusing discontent;
- encouraging organisation;
- nourishing good interpersonal relations;
- emphasising common objectives.

The worker helps the group to function by contributing calmness and objectivity, a focus on common goals and an 'analysis and treatment of the causes of tension to the degree that he and the group are able to handle them'.

Ross suggests that the contribution of the worker towards group development is not limited to being helpful in times of crises, disputes and various other blocks to cooperative work. The contribution is essentially ongoing and creative and at its best will help to foresee impending problems and avoid the need for crisis intervention. The nature of this continuing contribution is described by Ross in the following passage:

> The professional worker seeks also to increase the amount of satisfaction in interpersonal relations and in cooperative work. He is a warming, congenial influence in group and community meetings. This implies a warm, friendly person, sensitive to the deeper feelings of people, and interested in the 'little things' that are important in the lives of individuals and communities. He is concerned with meetings in which people feel comfortable, enjoy themselves and feel free to verbalise. To this end he is alert not only to the physical and psychological conditions which make for such comfort, but seeks to create these conditions and uses his own self to facilitate these. This means he is adept not only in room arrangements, introductions, casual conversations, but that he is sensitive to the process of interaction which goes on in a group and knows when and how to ask that question which will catch and focus the interest of the group, when to interpret what is being attempted, when to praise. People can enjoy working together when they begin to know one another and sense what they can do co-operatively. Part of the worker's role is to assure such satisfaction for the group.
>
> (Ross, 1967)

Ross' chapter on the role of the professional worker is a valuable contribution to our understanding of the tasks of the worker with local groups. Unfortunately, Ross tends to convey a picture of the neighbourhood worker as an angelic figure, moving with ease through the urban 'interpersonal underworld', suffusing it with light, reason and goodwill. It is this flavour in his book that often deterred readers from attending to what is probably one of the clearest expositions of those aspects of role that are concerned with the social and emotional needs of a group.

Another view of group maintenance pays attention to the task rather than the socio-emotional elements of group life; the major concern for the worker is with how the group functions as a work and decision-making system. The worker is interested in the effectiveness of the leaders of the group, its levels of participation and recruitment, and the extent to which it is representative of its constituency. The worker is most often seen as a 'resource and information person', feeding the group concrete data and resources, rather than more intangible assistance with, for example, disruptive aspects of the group dynamic.

Education in its broadest sense is at the heart of the work in group maintenance, and provides the final dimension that we wish to discuss in this brief introduction. We have referred already in this book to the distinction between *outcome* and *process* goals. The former refer to the end results of a group's activities, and the latter to the educative aspects of work through which both the group and individual members acquire competence and confidence in a number of skill and knowledge areas. The development of a group, and the learning and change that occur in individuals, are naturally not confined to those tasks that are to do with group maintenance; nevertheless, it is the task of group maintenance that provides by far the greatest challenge and opportunities for learning, and it is thus appropriate to refer to the educative aspects of involvement in community action in this chapter.

There is a variety of ways in which process goals are described. For example, some theorists and practitioners are essentially concerned with the development of knowledge and skills in those activities that need to be carried out if the group is to function effectively and achieve its goals. This will be more fully discussed later in the chapter, and they include the development of leadership potential, skills in negotiating and bargaining, and competence in tasks such as running meetings, keeping minutes and accounts, planning and the execution of group decisions. It is also expected that, as individuals learn and extend their skills, they will acquire more confidence in themselves, and there will be a development of the individual's personality, experience and life goals. This may be made manifest not only through the activities of the group but also in the individual's relationships and achievements in settings such as his or her family and work.

There are differences between writers and between practitioners in the importance that they give to that development of individuals that occurs *over and above the enhancement of those skills needed for task performance in the group*. The Biddles, for instance, give emphasis to the development of the whole individual; they see community work as a 'group method for expediting personality growth'. This view of community work – which Khinduka (1975) criticises as the psychological approach to social problems used essentially by caseworkers practising in a community setting – is also reflected in those schemes for participation that emphasise the therapeutic aspects of participation rather than the instrumental ones that give value to the social and political benefits of influencing decisions, achieving change and sharing power.

A different approach to individual change is one that gives most priority to the development of those skills that are needed to push forward the work of the group, and that give the individual the confidence and competence eventually to take part in wider community and city-wide issues. Neighbourhood workers who take this line accept that changes also occur that usually benefit the individual in his or her relations in the family and at work, but these changes are seen as 'spin-offs' that are to be welcomed but are not to be given priority, do not provide the basic rationale for neighbourhood work and should never impede the work of the group in achieving its goals. People do change as a result of being involved in community action, but such changes are ultimately valued because they facilitate, rather than justify, the work of the neighbourhood group. This is the approach of most capacity building and training programmes targeted at local residents.

We end this discussion by referring to those conceptions of process goals that tend to use the language of 'consciousness-raising'. The vocabulary of this view of process is that of enhancing political awareness, and the raising of consciousness, so that people become better able to understand and question those factors that perpetuate poverty and powerlessness. The influence of Paulo Freire, especially his argument that critical reflection is essential for meaningful action, has been considerable in this area. It is articulated by Margaret Ledwith who brings together Freirian and feminist thinking:

> The process of liberation begins in dialogue, a critical encounter that enables people to speak their word and name the world . . . Dialogue is a mutual process of action and reflection, which engages with deeply personal experiences and the profoundly political structures that have shaped them. It is the beginning of

humanisation, becoming more fully human in the world. But a dialogue of equals cannot happen without humility and criticality on the part of the community worker.

(Ledwith, 2020: 171)

There are, not surprisingly, differences of emphasis. There are those in community work who would see local people's involvement in neighbourhood groups ultimately justified by gains to be made in political understanding; action at a neighbourhood level might be criticised for being divisive and parochial, but acceptable so long as it deepens participants' awareness of the political and economic predicament of the excluded and prepares them for some eventual systematic confrontation with powerholders. Community workers and projects holding this view would define the process of learning about politics and organising as more important than the achievement of specific goals.

A different emphasis is given by those who stress the value in its own right of neighbourhood action, and the importance to local people of short-term gains and resources. Political learning is then valued in so far as it facilitates the work of the group, and helps individuals become involved in issues and problems outside their community. Such an involvement might just as well be reflected in membership of local political parties and turn-out at government and trade union elections as in the development of a critical class, race or feminist consciousness. This position may imply a continuum of consciousness along which individuals may progress; the value of such progress is seen to lie primarily in the benefits to the work of the group rather than in the importance of political learning in its own right.

The significant points on this continuum include:

1   Awareness of the self and one's position and abilities to achieve some change. This includes the emergence of a motivation to seek change. We have already referred to such changes in the sections on reflection and vision in Chapter 6.
2   Awareness of the collective aspects of a problem, that is, there are other people going through a similar situation or experience.
3   Awareness, not just of the possibilities of collective action but also of the powerfulness of the efforts of a group as compared with those of individuals. Individuals begin to assess the costs and benefits to themselves and to the community of engaging in a cooperative struggle around a local issue.
4   Awareness of the political nature of decisions made in organisations such as local authorities, partnership boards and forums about resources, opportunities and power sharing. 'Political' is used here to refer to the process of negotiating and bargaining that occurs over the allocation of scarce resources, and involves the key people or departments seeking to gain control over resources and power. Discussions between, and decisions by, elected members are only one aspect of the political process that occurs within local authorities, partnerships and other organisations.
5   Awareness of how the interests and concerns of one's own group relate to those of other groups in the neighbourhood, local agencies, a city or society as a whole. This awareness may reflect a strategic need to form alliances with others in order to achieve change, or the realisation of the need to avoid a situation where groups are competing with each other for the limited resources for community development held by agencies.

Points 4 and 5 on the continuum seem together to define a state of 'community consciousness' in which people have a political awareness that is bounded by the issues of
concern in the local community. They come to see how their lives are affected by these
issues, and to understand the powerful grip that organisational bureaucracies have
on the lives of many individuals and families. In their book on London's East End,
Katharine Mumford and Anne Power explore why community spirit, built up over a
period of time, is so significant for families:

> Overwhelmingly they attach great importance to it, even when they feel it is miss-
> ing. They recognise its core elements as social contact and communication, infor-
> mal mutual aid and support. They see it as a way of overcoming social and racial
> barriers, breaking down isolation, making people feel more responsible and creat-
> ing a sense of security.
>
> (Mumford and Power, 2003: 55)

6   Awareness and interest in broader political and socio-economic issues, for exam-
      ple, in regional, national and global issues. Such awareness, notably about cli-
      mate change, may lead to a new or renewed feeling of responsibility that may be
      reflected in participation in activities like elections and membership of political
      groups and parties.
7   Awareness of the world that goes beyond an interest in wanting to know what
      is going on. The individual develops a critical appreciation of his or her position
      and that of his or her peers in society, and explores *causal* questions about the
      arrangements that govern matters like the distribution of income, wealth, oppor-
      tunities and power. There is an obvious link here with the theoretical literature on
      adult education, community development and transformative action.

Members of a neighbourhood work group will be at different stages on this continuum, each of which is worthy in its own right, and each of which contributes to
the work and potential of the group. The effect of this contribution need not necessarily be always helpful – a group may be deflected in its task both by new members
who are at the early stages of consciousness and by more 'experienced' members who
persist in raising 'fundamental' issues before the rest of the group is ready to deal with
them. The essential point is that it is certainly not necessary (though ideologists may
view it as desirable) for any of the members of a community group to develop more
'advanced' states of consciousness in order for that group to achieve its goals. Politically 'unaware' people do participate in groups that achieve much for their constituency and neighbourhood.

   We wish now to develop a more detailed account of the tasks that face the neighbourhood worker in helping to maintain and strengthen the community group. We
describe here the five major categories of activity of the worker. They are:

- providing resources and information;
- being supportive;
- coordinating help;
- planning;
- developing confidence and competence.

Providing resources and information

In order to carry out their work effectively, community groups need a variety of resources and a way of gathering and processing information. The worker is an important, but not the only, element in the provision of both resources and information. Ross has described this as the 'expert' role of the worker, providing data and direct advice in such areas as community diagnosis, research skills, information about other communities, advice on methods of organisation and procedure and technical information.

Providing resources

The word 'resources' has increasingly become a cover-all word and is used in a variety of ways to label a diversity of functions and activities. We use it to refer to the material facilities and aid that a worker can provide for a group. The worker may not be able directly to provide all such resources (nor think it desirable to do so) but will be a point of access or of information about them. The kinds of resources we have in mind include the following:

Basic resources

These are the essential tools that the group needs to do its work. These include secretarial and clerical help, telephone, computer, notepaper, photocopier, files, records and overhead projector. In addition to these, a group may need from time to time resources like transport and equipment for specific events such as jumble sales, meetings and parties.

Accommodation

The group will need a space for committee and group meetings, for holding events and for running particular services, for example, a weekly advice and information surgery. The matter of premises was discussed in Chapter 7.

Money

The budget will need to be enough to finance the day-to-day costs of the group's work, and also any special projects it wishes to run such as a summer playscheme. The worker may not only advise on where to obtain funds but also be a point of access to sources of funds in local agencies as well as funding provided by government programmes and trusts Some workers can also access 'seed money' within their organisations with which to help the setting up of groups.

People

Most community groups will require volunteers to take part in specific activities; and specialists (e.g. lawyers) to advise them on certain aspects of their work. Other kinds of specialists might also be needed, such as local craftspeople, to carry out some work for the group, and celebrities to open a group function such as a community fair.

Special resources

On some occasions, special equipment will be needed for one-off tasks, for example, a camcorder, a colour printer and tape recorders.

Providing information

The kinds of information that the neighbourhood worker provides or helps in providing may be seen to consist of the following:

Basic information

The range of such information is wide. It includes that considered above relating to resources as well as data on, for example, local agencies, facts and figures on the neighbourhood, and on substantive areas of knowledge in fields such as economic development, housing and environment, planning and welfare rights. It also includes information on matters such as keeping accounts, preparing a press statement, opening a bank account and keeping minutes. It is extremely difficult to convey the scope of the information that most workers will be called upon to give, or know where to find. The availability of websites, which contain much of the information being sought, is mainstream in neighbourhood work, in terms of both workers making use of the technology and of them encouraging groups to do the same.

- *General advice.* Here the worker helps in advising on the pros and cons of various issues and courses of action, and in predicting the costs, benefits and general outcomes of matters like new legislation, decisions and events that affect the work of the group. The worker might advise, for example, on the effects of new arrangements for the submission of funding applications or on a change a group wants to make in its constitution, or on whether it should register as a charity. The worker's advice is sought and given, but she does not expect it to have a special status in the group and it must be considered alongside that of other members.
- *Interpretation and analysis.* There is often a role for the worker in helping a group to understand the details and implications of, for example, various proposals and documents such as planning applications and new legislation, as well as 'difficult' letters from officers in large organisations that are full of jargon, unfamiliar language, style and vagueness.

In general, the worker has to consider the presentation of information in terms of how much is given, its timing, its form and style, the medium through which it is conveyed, the characteristics of the people who want it, and the use to which it will be put by them.

The reader might consider, for example, how one would take these factors into account in responding to a request from a newly formed tenants' association in a tower block 'for a couple of model constitutions'.

The task of providing information and resources appears straightforward, although demanding a good deal of the worker's time, skills and integrity. It is, however, not without its pitfalls. There are the two related issues of learning and control. It is in the role of information giver that workers most frequently experience the dilemma of how helpful they should be to a group. If, for example, a group wants a list of local authority committee chairpersons, the worker might suffer considerable anguish in deciding whether to provide it herself (the quickest solution) or work with members of the group in getting hold of the information (longer, but adds a little to the skill and knowledge of the group).

The other dilemma occurs because of the association of information with power and control. Through the selective withholding and giving of information, a neighbourhood worker can unfortunately create opportunities to influence the work of a group. The worker may have the best motives in doing so; she or he may be right in assessing that a certain piece of information would only distract the group from its task. But the worker may be aware that to withhold the information is also to withhold the opportunity for the group to decide on its relevance, and thus to undermine its authority.

Finally, we wish briefly to mention a further problematic aspect of the role of information/resource person. It is that the role offers the opportunity to the worker to establish herself or himself as a go-between, mediating between the group and other organisations and decision makers in the local authority. Even if the worker does not take these opportunities, involvement in information exchange may lead to the worker being perceived and responded to as a go-between. The role of go-between is, of course, a recognised one in community work though it is also rejected as being inappropriate by many workers on the grounds that it diminishes the responsibility and authority of the group. It should not be confused with the go-between role of key residents, discussed in Chapter 6, to facilitate the early work of the neighbourhood worker.

Being supportive

Another of the neighbourhood worker's tasks is to be supportive both of the group and of its individual members. The group particularly needs the support and encouragement of the worker at times when its energies and enthusiasm are low, and it feels it has suffered setbacks, or achieved little, in reaching its goals. The worker can often be supportive at such times by maintaining the interest, optimism and commitment that seem to be waning in group members. She attempts to re-galvanise and re-motivate participants. But support of the group should also be ongoing, and the worker can provide it by indicating his or her recognition and respect of its work.

Support for the group is also given when the worker helps its members to assess and evaluate its work, assisting them to see the positive and creative aspects of what they have done. It is given, too, by the worker ably carrying out the work she has offered, or been requested, to do on behalf of the group, by attendance and helpfulness at its meetings and neighbourhood events, by 'mucking-in' and taking a share of the routine and boring side of the group's activities, and by being a figure of continuity during those periods when the group is going through changes associated with the loss or the recruitment of members.

There are a number of ways in which the worker gives support to *individuals* of a community group through, for instance, being supportive of individuals' learning and experimenting in new roles, such as chair or treasurer, and of those learning new and challenging tasks. The worker will help individuals to develop their feelings of competence about new roles and tasks, and confirm their sense of how they contribute to the work of the group. Some members of a group might also expect the worker to help them to assess the costs and benefits of their remaining involved in collective action, discussing, for example, the amount of help or opposition they are experiencing from family or close neighbours. Such support could as much involve helping individuals to find a way of leaving a group as supporting them to persevere.

In this respect, it is important to note that some individuals may call upon the worker for support and advice about problems in their family or work, or with agencies like the police and the courts. This support may be very tangible indeed, such as asking the worker to stand bail or act as a guarantor to a hire purchase agreement. It is not necessarily only problems with which the worker may be approached; her support may be needed for new endeavours that a person wants to undertake, not just in the work of the group but also in the person's job or in some other aspect of community life.

The style in which workers undertake tasks may also be seen to constitute a source of support to local people. Friendliness, openness and a willingness to be available for a discussion, even during the hard-pressed moments of a hectic day, can contribute support and encouragement. It is evident in the relationships of many workers to community groups that the support can be a two-way affair. Workers may value the opportunity for discussing work matters with local people, or opportunities that are likely to occur in their personal or work lives. In particular, residents may offer feedback to the worker about how he or she relates to them, and about the way in which the worker goes about the job. Residents can offer, too, more general support to the worker as they relate to each other in different roles in perhaps less familiar settings, such as a mosque or a sports stadium.

Workers need to be cautious here because of the issues to do with confidentiality, dependency and 'inappropriate' friendships. This should not mean, however, that the possibility of reciprocity should be ignored. Our experience is that both residents and workers appreciate, often with hindsight, the support they receive from each other. The combination of friendship, an element of dependency and mutual learning can be a rich outcome of community development that deserves to be given more attention.

Coordinating help

No neighbourhood group is, or ought to be, an island unto itself. Groups which are actively engaged in community action, and which want to achieve their goals, will have developed a host of relationships with other groups, individuals, local government, partnerships, health and voluntary agencies as well as community institutions such as schools, churches, trades unions, and civic and political bodies. Many of these relationships develop because they provide access to resources and information that the community group needs in its work. A more detailed examination of these external affairs of a group is provided in the next chapter.

The worker has an important role not just in facilitating knowledge of, or access to, these external resources but also in helping to coordinate their contribution to the work of the community group. Without some planning and coordination of the help provided by 'outside' people, a community group may be as much at risk of being hindered and deflected by external help as assisted by it.

These 'outsiders' are often referred to as 'experts' or 'specialists' brought in by the group to assist with limited and one-off aspects of its work. The Biddles have described this concern of the worker as helping the group to use expert resources without surrendering to them. Many community groups battling with complex issues in fields such as transport, environment and crime prevention often need competent legal and technical advice. Occasionally they may receive a grant that enables them to pay for this advice, but normally they will need to seek out specialists who are sympathetic to their interests and who will provide their time and advice for little or no payment. Community groups operating in the vicinity of a university or college may attract the interest of students or staff members who have, or who are acquiring, the special expertise required by the group.

The use of outside specialists is not without its costs. So much depends on their ability to 'demystify' their expertise and to present their advice to the group in ways which its members can understand and use. Specialists, especially those brought in to advise the group on a one-off basis, can unwittingly confuse and undermine group members by the abstractions and detail of their advice, by the way in which it is presented and by the personal manner and style of the advice givers. Experts can too easily succumb to feelings of wanting 'to take the group by the scruff of its neck' where they believe the group is going about things in the wrong way, or too slowly. They may not appreciate or understand the neighbourhood worker's concern that group members have the opportunity to make their own decisions, and to carry them out themselves. Outside specialists may need to be helped to shift away from seeing the group as a 'client' and to perceive the nature of their contribution as a collaborative one. This can often open up useful training and education opportunities, including joint training between residents, practitioners and managers.

The potential for a neighbourhood worker to be involved directly in training for community members is widely acknowledged – he or she becomes the outside specialist. Sarah Banks describes how a community worker (Joan) on an estate trained as a tutor and co-facilitated a 10-week 'Learning about community work' course. It recruited a mixture of 13 residents and regeneration/community workers from the estate and elsewhere:

> Joan felt that the success of the course in engaging interest and motivation of local people was due to the fact that it was held in the centre, it focused on issues and skills of immediate relevance and she was a tutor. As she commented: 'Because I was doing it, it was safe, because I'd built up relationships with the people'.
>
> (Banks, 2007: 91)

The activity of the neighbourhood worker in coordinating the help of outside experts may be conceptualised in the following way:

1 Anticipating the needs of a group for specialist help, being able to locate experts and assisting the group to interest them in the work of the group.
2 Helping group members to make the best use of the specialists by providing information on them and their agencies, clarifying as precisely as possible the issues about which advice is needed, and encouraging group members to adopt a questioning or critical stance towards experts.
3 Familiarising the specialists with the composition, procedures, goals and history of the group, and with the nature of the neighbourhood in which it operates. This

may be partly achieved if the group provides access for the specialists to its files and records, but it is just as important for the specialist to 'tune in' to the neighbourhood and the group in informal social settings.

4 Advising the specialists about their role in the group and drawing their attention to any negative consequences that their contribution may be having. The worker and the group will want to ensure that specialists do not come to dominate, and that the group does not become overdependent on their advice. The authority of group members may gradually and imperceptibly wither in the face of the specialists' knowledge of their subjects and the issues confronting the group, or in the face of the enthusiasm, energies and single-mindedness of outsiders like students.

5 'Translating' the advice of the specialists for group members. No matter how well advice has been presented, the worker may need to continue to work with members after the group's meetings in order to better understand and clarify the contribution of the specialists, and to assess the implications of that advice for the work of the group and the support of its constituency.

6 Keeping the specialists 'on ice' so that they are ready to respond to the group when it approaches them. This involves the worker in keeping them informed of the work of the group, and securing their continued interest in its affairs. This can be done by the group inviting them to its social occasions and to activities like fund-raising events and annual general meetings. There is a particular role for the worker in securing the continued support of outside helpers when the worker has left the group. This is discussed in Chapter 11.

The task of the neighbourhood worker in coordinating outside help does not necessarily imply a role of 'go-between' or intermediary. On the contrary, the task of the worker is not to stand as a filter or channel between the group and outside helpers but rather to promote direct and personal contact between them. The worker's responsibility is to make this direct contact as fruitful as possible, and thus to ensure that the use of specialists has a positive impact on the work of the group. The worker's interest in facilitating the interaction between group and external helpers is to see that group members enhance their own confidence and abilities in finding and using such help. The worker aims for a point in group development where his role in facilitating this interaction becomes less significant.

Planning

It may at first appear incongruous to separate out planning as an activity. It has been an essential aspect of many of the worker's and group's activities that have been discussed in this book.

In Chapters 3 and 5, for example, we considered the planning of the neighbourhood worker's entry and subsequent interventions in a neighbourhood. In Chapter 4 we stressed the importance of planning in carrying out a collection of data about a neighbourhood. We have also drawn attention to the value of planning for events like meetings and deputations.

We have identified it here as a separate activity largely because effective planning – a concern to anticipate and prepare for future events, and to initiate them – is essential to the maintenance of a soundly functioning and successful organisation. This is particularly the case for neighbourhood groups where a number of factors may conspire to make them over-involved in their present activities and less concerned with what the future holds for them and their constituency. For instance, most residents participate in neighbourhood groups in their spare time; they may only have the energy to interest themselves with the immediate concerns of a group, and insufficient energy to enable them to plan ahead. Immediate issues may be so pressing and complex and a group's resources so inadequate that group members are forced to attend to things as and when they happen. In this way, there is often a tendency for neighbourhood groups to do things incrementally, and to be reactive to events in their community and to the requirements of their own operations.

There appears to be a role for the worker in promoting a concern in the neighbourhood group with two kinds of planning: policy and operations.

Policy planning

Here the planning is to do with the salient issues and problems facing a group's constituency or the community of which it is a part. This kind of planning will concern some neighbourhood groups more than others. For example, a group set up to oppose the speculative redevelopment of an area, or one set up to deal with employment opportunities, will find it essential to forecast and predict major policy decisions and shifts, and to identify trends in the demography and work patterns of the working and resident population of the neighbourhood. Such a group may wish to initiate discussion of future issues and events that may not yet have been considered by policymakers or the general public. Indeed, groups should be encouraged to be pro-active in their discussions, not just responding to, for example, consultations about proposals but putting forward alternative ideas.

Operations planning

All neighbourhood groups must attend to this kind of planning if they are to survive and be successful. Operations planning is to do with the group's own administrative and political procedures. It consists of the following six concerns:

1   The setting of goals and priorities based on evidence as well as aspirations.
2   Identifying, acquiring and planning the use of resources within and outside the group so as best to achieve the group's goals
3   A rational process of dividing up work and allocating responsibilities.
4   Administering and coordinating the various sub-groups and activities that comprise the neighbourhood group
5   Devising and keeping to procedures to ensure that tasks are completed and deadlines met. This involves planning the preparation and submission of, for example, reports to sponsors, applications for funding, petitions to policy-makers and information to constituents. It also involves the kind of detailed planning that is necessary to mount a successful community event such as a festival.
6   Preparing the group's tactics and strategies in its negotiations with decision makers. This comprises discussing which available tactics are feasible and desirable for the task in hand, evaluating their costs and benefits to the group and trying to assess the likely consequences of particular courses of action.

A word of caution is necessary here. It is not suggested that workers impose planning tasks or frameworks on to groups; rather, they should first listen and observe in order to see any less obvious ways in which a group may be engaged in planning its affairs, for example, in informal conversations amongst key players outside meetings.

Developing confidence and competence

One of the neighbourhood worker's fundamental concerns from the very outset of contacts with local people is to help them acquire confidence and competence in themselves and their abilities to carry out tasks on behalf of the group. We have highlighted this aspect of the work within the central part of our account of the process of neighbourhood work for two reasons: because the maintenance of the group is dependent upon carrying out a variety of activities and because the neighbourhood worker will find that a large proportion of his or her time, energies and skill is needed to help people develop their abilities in the kinds of tasks outlined in the following. The availability of accredited training courses and the involvement of local people in evaluating and analysing community projects are indications of the importance now attached to this aspect of neighbourhood work.

The practitioner has the job of helping local people acquire confidence and competence in two broad categories of tasks – the technical and the interactional. We shall consider each separately, though in practice they are intimately connected and often difficult to distinguish.

Technical tasks

These tasks are often referred to as civic or committee skills. They comprise a wide range of jobs involved in the administration of the affairs of the community group. Lower order technical tasks that have to be carried out in most groups include writing emails and letters, keeping accounts, preparing agendas, taking minutes and using the telephone as well as other items such as maintaining computers, photocopiers and video equipment, and printing and distributing newsletters. Higher order tasks include matters such as carrying out a community audit, organising a petition, leading a deputation, appearing on television and local radio, giving a conference presentation and challenging the ways in which services are provided by the local authority, health and other agencies. Increasingly, groups will need to plan for how they use social media and maintain websites as forums for local bulletin boards, debates etc.

We must stress that these are only examples; the nature of the technical tasks will vary with the concerns and issues facing particular groups. But whatever the nature of these tasks, the neighbourhood worker will be heavily engaged in helping people to develop sufficient skills and knowledge to accomplish them.

We are hesitant to use the terms lower and higher order technical tasks because we do not wish to imply that the higher order tasks are necessarily more difficult. The contrary is often the case: neighbourhood workers will frequently find themselves spending time encouraging people in tasks like writing emails or managing finances. It will depend on the experience of individual members of each group whether the lower order tasks are easily accomplished. The time spent by the worker in helping with tasks like writing minutes and funding applications will vary with the experience and background of the individuals concerned. The worker who has spent several hours helping a secretary do the letters that have resulted from the previous evening's committee meeting will often feel very tempted to do the work herself in order to have done with it quickly. A worker who is doing the job properly can at least expect the time put in on such work to begin to diminish as group members become more skilled and confident.

Although the general rule is that the worker's job is to encourage group members to do the work, there will clearly be some exceptional occasions when the worker finds that she has to do some of the technical tasks herself. Such occasions occur, for example, if the relevant group officer is ill or not functioning in the group because of, say, domestic or work problems. Emergencies often occur, for example, when a group has a week's notice to submit a funding application, and the need for the worker actively to assist in the production of the application will override any considerations for the learning of group members.

Interactional tasks

Interactional tasks are of two kinds: political skills and competence, and caring and supportive capacities within the neighbourhood group.

Group members need to become adept in political transactions within the group, and between the group and the constituency that it represents. The group also has to develop skills in managing its relationships with organisations in its environment – the town hall, partnership bodies, service agencies, potential resource people and groups, the press and television, other neighbourhood groups, councillors, MPs, trade unions, and public and private industries. Groups need to be particularly alert to the danger of being controlled or manipulated by councillors and be confident about clarifying the amount of involvement of councillors. Relationships with all these systems require broad political skills in representing, and negotiating for, the interests of the group. It also includes competence in executing and evaluating chosen strategies and tactics.

People who take leadership roles in neighbourhood groups also need to care for the emotional life of the group, and to be aware of how events in people's personal lives affect the group's work. Caring for the group also involves 'training' members for leadership roles, sharing the burden of the work and attending to the recruitment of new members. The neighbourhood worker and leaders need to understand, and mobilise in the group's interest, the original and changing motivations for membership of the group, and to be sensitive to the effect of behaviour in the group like scapegoating. It is clear that the 'caring' aspects of these interactional tasks encompass many of the points discussed earlier in this chapter in the section called 'Being supportive', and that there is often a connection between group accomplishment and group members' development. Successful action can often pull people out of their personal antagonisms.

One difficulty in looking at interactional skills from the point of view of individual members is that it may distract our attention away from the group as a system. Groups take on a life and a force of their own that is something more than that given to it by the sum contribution of its individual members.

The theories or models of group change that a worker will use to understand what is going on in a group, and the phases through which it is proceeding, will be determined by a number of factors, not least of which will be their proven usefulness to the worker in helping in her work. No one way of conceptualising group development is necessarily better or more correct than another. It may be that workers will need to draw upon a variety of explanations about group behaviour according to how they best explain the phenomena present in a group at a particular time.

Groups change and develop, and it is part of the neighbourhood worker's role to help group members understand that these changes are taking place, and to appreciate their effect on the way individuals are relating to one another and contributing to the work of the group. Many workers are understandably suspicious about including a concern with group development and dynamics as part of their work. We stress that the role of the worker is 'to keep an eye on what is happening' and to assist group members to understand and respond to the nature of group change and processes. It is not suggested that the worker intervenes to bring about substantial changes in the group's life, even if it were possible for her, as a single individual, to do so.

The job of helping people develop skills in technical and interactional tasks demands of the worker time and patience. The availability of time to allow her to work with group members on these tasks is in turn a product of the worker's own ability to manage the workload and not to be so overburdened that she is unable to find the space to sit down with a group member to help with the tasks which need to be carried out. Developing the technical and interactional skills of a group also demands flexibility of the worker in the kind of role she is prepared to take on.

There will be occasions in the life of a group when its maintenance will hinge on whether the worker is prepared to accept a role (e.g. the post of treasurer) that she would not normally want to have. Another kind of flexibility is that of being able to take on 'missing roles' in the group. The worker may become aware that the work of the group is being hindered because there is no one in the group helping the less confident members to participate, or no one who is clarifying and summarising the points of a discussion as it proceeds. The kind of roles that the worker may temporarily fill, and model for group members were discussed in Chapter 5 in relation to non-directive role behaviour.

Equal opportunities

It is essential for the worker to keep the issue of equal opportunities on a group's agenda. A community group may assume that they are inclusive, stating that they are open to anyone living in the neighbourhood, when in reality a variety of people may feel they cannot become involved – because, for instance, they are disabled or black. The Equality Act 2010 consolidates a number of discrimination laws into a single statute. Neighbourhood workers need to be familiar with the main elements of the legislation without necessarily being experts. Their main contribution will be through their practice, in how they work with groups to raise awareness of discrimination and seek to overcome barriers, encouraging group members to actively and willingly engage with equality issues. Two ways of ensuring that the issue does not get lost is for the worker to intervene by (a) *asking questions,* for example, who else lives round here? What percentage of the population consists of people from minority ethnic groups? How many new members have joined the community group over the last year? and (b) *providing checklists* in relation to particular aspects of the group's work.

However, the key to encouraging a group to address the question of equal opportunities will lie chiefly in *how* the worker raises it with a group – it will require the worker to use tact and sensitivity while at the same time conveying clearly and firmly the essential value base of equal opportunities. Achieving this balance will be facilitated if the worker already has a good working relationship with the group.

What a worker has to do to keep the organisation going is partly dependent on what happens to the group in its relationship with other organisations. We started this chapter by suggesting that the way in which 'they', the authorities, respond can critically affect the stability and confidence of a group. In the next chapter we want to look more closely at what is involved for a worker in helping a group in its relationships with organisations such as local partnerships and federations.

References

Banks, S. (2007) 'Working in and with community groups and organisations: processes and practice' in H. Butcher *et al*. (eds) *Critical community practice*, Bristol: The Policy Press.

Barr, A. (1977) *The practice of neighbourhood community work*, York: Department of Social Administration and Social Work, University of York.

Brager, G. and Specht, H. (1973) *Community organising*, New York: Columbia University Press.

Khinduka, S. K. (1975) 'Community development: potential and limitations', in R. Kramer and H. Specht (eds) *Readings in community organisation practice* (2nd edn), Englewood Cliffs, NJ: Prentice-Hall.

Ledwith, M. (2020) *Community development. A critical approach* (3rd edn), Bristol: The Policy Press.

Mumford, K. and Power, A. (2003) *East enders. Faith and community in East London*, Bristol: The Policy Press.

Ross, M. (1967) *Community organisation* (2nd edn), London: Harper & Row.

10 Dealing with friends and enemies

A delegation from an active tenants' association on a large estate of some 2,500 dwellings meets with members/staff of a local charitable trust.

The tenants are accompanied by a neighbourhood worker who is responsible for a wider area than the tenants' estate. She is there to support their application to the trust for a grant which will enable them to employ a neighbourhood worker who would work only on their estate.

The purpose of today's meeting is for the trust to obtain a clearer idea of the proposed job, before it reaches a decision on the application. It wants to know, specifically, what the neighbourhood worker would do; that is, the trust wants to acquire a better understanding of the roles, tasks and skills involved in doing neighbourhood work. It is also anxious to know why the present neighbourhood worker cannot continue to serve the estate in addition to the larger area.

This is a briefing for a role play exercise we have used during training workshops for neighbourhood workers. In addition to testing the ability of workers to articulate what it is they do in neighbourhood work, the role play also forces workers to examine the question of how a community group relates to other groups and organisations in the community. The material focuses on the issue of the planning, tactics and techniques that a group can practise and adopt in order to achieve its objectives; in this example it has to know what the meeting is about, find out who is on the trust committee, send them papers in advance, decide who in the delegation is to speak on particular issues and how best to present the argument. It also has to know what role the neighbourhood worker will play in the meeting.

Giving attention to these kinds of detailed practice questions flows from an examination of the theme of the 'external affairs' of a group, of how it relates to both

DOI: 10.4324/9781003310006-10

friendly and hostile elements of society with which it comes into contact. We shall explore four components of this:

- identifying and negotiating with decision makers;
- a group's relationship to other groups and organisations in the community;
- a group's own constituency and the general public;
- the social policy perspective – city, regional, national and global issues.

A group that has become skilled in its relationship to other systems will often be in a position of having to manage significant financial and human resources. In the final section of this chapter, we discuss how the administration and provision of resources or services appear to demand particular skills.

Identifying and negotiating with decision makers

Action by community groups and neighbourhood workers which relates to influencing decision-making processes must necessarily draw upon substantial political skills. While knowledge of political and administrative studies is an essential part of neighbourhood workers' training, they need to relate closely to the kinds of issues which are likely to confront neighbourhood groups. An intellectual understanding of political processes has to be combined with practical political skills. We shall see how the ability to 'read a political situation', to think and act politically, are essential prerequisites for a community group and a neighbourhood worker. Without them, neither group nor worker is likely to be effective over time. Nor will their survival chances be high. It is possible to distinguish three contexts of community action where the political skills of identifying and negotiating with decision makers are of paramount importance.

Building a profile of the target

Whether a group is to have a low-key exchange of opinions with a decision-making body or a tough dialogue over a particular issue, it needs to put time and energy into finding out about that particular organisation: what resources does it have, what is its mandate, what new ideas is it interested in, who does it represent, how is it controlled, what is its constituency? These are broad strategic questions which can be applied to most organisations and a neighbourhood worker can encourage a group to consider them.

Clearly, the worker can share with a group the information he collects when constructing organisational profiles, which we discussed in Chapter 4.

However, the most pointed questions are usually about where power, authority and influence within an organisation lie. Locating these will help a group to present a case, to win allies or to achieve change. The Carnegie UK Trust has published a guide for groups and organisations which want to explore power in relation to achieving change (Hunjan and Pettit, 2011). Paul Bunyan, in an article on broad-based organising, makes the case for the reassertion of political activity in community development (Bunyan, 2010).

Two important factors for a worker to consider when deciding what change he hopes to achieve within an organisation are:

- an organisation's decision-making process – who is likely to exercise both formal authority and informal influence on the outcome of a proposal. In other words, how decisions are made and who is in a position to influence the process;
- whether those who exercise formal authority or informal influence in the decision-making process are likely to agree or disagree with a proposal. This kind of analysis is important because it enables a worker and group to anticipate how much resistance or support a proposal is likely to meet.

A community group which 'sizes up' an organisation in this way is likely to be in a far stronger strategic and tactical position than the group which neglects to do so. The neighbourhood worker can play a crucial role here, especially by raising appropriate questions with the leadership of a group. The approach must include an attempt to anticipate what effects a group's action will have: 'Whether educating, bargaining, or disrupting, community workers and groups must assess what response or retaliation is possible from the target as they plan their course of action' (Brager and Specht, 1973). Such an assessment can best be made through a concerted and planned effort to find out about and understand the target group. Fiona Ballantyne provides an example of how an umbrella group for community councils in part of Scotland was helped by a community worker to analyse a situation from all angles:

> There was discontent rising within several communities. At the same time the local authority was experiencing a bombardment of policy initiatives and directives from central government and was interested in obtaining support from a cross-section of interests. The worker encouraged the umbrella group to view the local authority as seeking 'friends,' pointing out that the organisation could fulfil this role whilst also pursuing a key place at the decision-making table.
>
> (Ballantyne, personal communication)

Negotiating by community groups

Community groups inevitably use up considerable time and energy in negotiating with decision-making organisations. Usually negotiation takes the form of bargaining between a group and an organisation. Negotiating can usefully be seen as a process in itself, rather than approximating to a once-and-for-all event. For example, an invitation by a group to members of a trust to visit it could be made months before an application for funds was submitted, yet the visit could influence the outcome of the application.

Two essential pre-negotiating tasks for a group are detailed preparation of a negotiating stance and practice or rehearsal of the case to be put. If a delegation is due to go into a negotiating meeting, the roles of its members have to be agreed upon in advance: who will outline the background to the issue, who will supply factual information, who will articulate the group's case, who will respond to offers made across the table?

Having decided upon the orchestration of their negotiation, members of the delegation should be encouraged to rehearse it: entering the room, introducing themselves, re-arranging the seating to their advantage, working out a signal to request an adjournment during the meeting.

If the idea of anticipating and practising in this way appears excessive, it should be remembered that negotiating is not only one of the most significant actions for a group but also often one where it can be most vulnerable. Powerful agencies can outwit, co-opt or outlast a community group in a protracted negotiating process, and the experiences of many groups tell a similar story. Preparation and practice can offset the power imbalance to some extent, and give leaders of a group or a delegation critical confidence and competence. Brager and Specht select three priority skills in negotiating by community groups:

Formulating demands: The outcome of bargaining is determined by the way in which demands are formulated rather than by the merits of the case or by the pressures applied during bargaining.

Regulating threat: Threats may be communicated with varying degrees of firmness.

*Reasonableness vs obstinacy:*Reasonableness suggests that a settlement is possible; obstinacy implies that real concessions must be made. This is why negotiating teams sometimes embody both approaches in different team members.

(Brager and Specht, 1973)

Community groups can become very skilled at negotiating, including being able to end up on occasions with a 'win-win' situation rather than one which is won for one party and lost for the other. The potential for a 'win-win' outcome can be seen increasingly in sustainable development projects. It is also evident in community development approaches to conflict resolution, particularly in post-conflict societies such as South Africa and Northern Ireland (see O'Brien, 2007).

Deciding strategy

In our experience, community groups in the past have tended to operate with a relatively simple strategic framework. This may have reflected a preference for a pragmatic approach, as well as a tendency for community projects to be composed of a range of interests and political views. Their framework was often expressed in terms of choosing either consensus or conflict strategies. However, there is evidence of groups using more complex typologies, such as the one advanced by Brager and Specht (1973) (quoted earlier).

Groups carry out effective strategic action in relation to target organisations, but we suggest that they tend to do so implicitly, rather than by making explicit use of the language of strategy building, whether this be influenced by social psychology or political science. The following questions are central to that process.

What will the outcome be?

Groups need to be clear about the desired end result of a strategy. In the case of seeking funds, for example, will public or private funding be most appropriate? There is little point in a group engaging in an exhausting struggle for government funding if it is clear that the conditions under which a grant is made will be unacceptable and that they cannot be changed.

Equally, a group needs to consider the implications of allowing its strategy to depend too much on one or two external individuals, in case the same people retain their grip on the group's future once they have helped it achieve a particular goal. We take an example from Orebro, a medium-sized town in Sweden where the city council, under the leadership of its deputy mayor, made a major commitment to developing democratic models throughout the local authority and among citizen groups:

Orebro – The Citizens City

A programme for the development of local democracy

- We want a deepening democracy with more people taking part in decision-making.
- People sharing influence and responsibility are conditions for a good society.
- As many citizens as possible shall have the opportunity to discuss and work together with the elected representatives and staff.
- Planning and decision-making should be looked upon as a dialogue in which everyone can learn from each other.
- Dialogue takes time but creates a strong democracy – a participatory democracy.

(CESAM/SABO, 2000)

Such a manifesto is music to the ears of community groups. Our point, however, is that both they and neighbourhood workers need to be alert to the danger of becoming too dependent on the enthusiasm of one or two well-placed, committed individuals. A group is wise to look ahead at the possible outcomes of making major use of a strong ally, and weigh up the advantages and disadvantages.

Which tactics?

A group needs to select the direction of its strategy and then proceed to weave together tactics which support it. Most groups employ both 'inside' and 'outside' tactics, obtaining results by both having allies inside large bureaucratic organisations and making their presence felt by clever use of resources external to the target organisation – effective publicity being especially important.

Who should be lobbied?

Related to the question of political tactics is that of the types of 'resource transaction' implied by an issue or problem: groups, for example, may wish to acquire a certain resource – a community centre, open space, a van – or they may seek to improve the quality of existing resources or services – caretaking facilities, a playground, surgery opening hours. We develop this typology of resource transactions at the end of the chapter. Here we alert the reader to the point that the nature of a neighbourhood worker's support of a group needs to be influenced by the type of transaction being planned by it, because certain transactions are likely to require particular personal qualities, attributes and skills.

Opinions voiced by community groups will not be heard by target organisations unless they are presented to influential people in these organisations convincingly and forcefully. The former requires there to be good, linked arguments, supported with valid evidence; the latter requires groups to lobby. Deciding who to talk to, and how best to arrange to do so, can pay dividends in terms of the ability of community groups to achieve their goals.

It is important that lobbying is perceived neither as a last-minute effort nor as a sufficient tactic by itself, for then the person or persons being lobbied will feel themselves to be under unacceptable pressures and will also tend to regard those who are doing the lobbying as motivated chiefly by self-interest. If a group has relied for support on one political party in the town hall and made no effort to communicate with other parties, it cannot expect to be listened to by the latter if the group suddenly sees how they could be useful to it.

Lobbying consists of building trust and interest between a group and those with political influence, and this can be demanding on a group's time, patience and resources. Often it involves 'being around' when important meetings take place, and informal talk in canteens and bars. The times when it is possible for a group to do intensive lobbying on a particular issue are comparatively rare, and the effectiveness of such lobbying depends on strong connections having been built up beforehand. Lobbying is an established feature of Britain's political system, and there is no reason why community groups should not gain benefits from it. In attempting to do so, however, they should not underestimate the skills required.

What leverage do we have?

A stage beyond lobbying is when a group knows that it can bring to bear real threat on a target organisation, and when it is in the interest of that organisation to give in to threat. This is known as leverage. It implies that considerable work has gone into compiling a profile of an organisation, to the extent that its vulnerable areas have been discovered. The effective use of leverage depends upon accurate forecasting of an organisation's actions so that a group can bring about the desired response.

Probably the most frequent form of leverage deployed in neighbourhood work, associated with the tactics of Alinsky, is the use of embarrassment, which either exposes an agency to public ridicule or undermines the 'professionalism' of agency staff. Examples would be: peaceful demonstration on immaculate lawns surrounding municipal buildings by children demanding play areas; publicising the wealthy residence of a private landlord who refuses to undertake repairs and maintenance of his homes; and exposure of policy contradictions of an organisation through the release of confidential information.

As the last example suggests, making use of leverage tactics can place a group on a moral knife-edge, and any group needs to think carefully about both the ethics and the consequences of employing such tactics; the costs of using leverage can outweigh the benefits if a group is seen to be using manipulative means in public life, since it is these that community work values purport to oppose. And making use of leverage risks leaving a group more vulnerable than before. Leverage can be an ultimate test of how able a group is at gamesmanship when implementing its strategy. It has been used with varying degrees of success and validity by the community organising movement.

Is the timing right?

The most important strategic consideration of all for community groups concerns the timing of any action; in some cases this can be even more vital than which issue a group chooses, for skilful timing may have the potential for opening the way for several issues. In terms of having greatest impact on decision-making, a group must aim to become involved in the process as early as possible. Planning and housing issues in particular have to be confronted before authorities take crucial decisions which then allow for only minor modification. The difficulty with early involvement is that it puts a severe strain on the ability of groups to sustain an even level of commitment over a long time. We have noted already how groups tend to become increasingly vulnerable, in a negotiating process, to the pressures of better-resourced and more expert agencies.

The question of timing highlights the role of the neighbourhood worker as a significant source of support for groups as they search for effective strategies with which to influence decision makers. Taking the position of always acting as a resource to a group demands considerable self-discipline by the worker, well explored by Von Hoffman:

> The best organisers have single-track minds. They care only for building the organisation. When they alienate a potential member they do so out of organisational need, not out of the egotism of irrelevant personal values. The best organisers stifle their tastes, their opinions, and their private obsessions.
>
> (Von Hoffman, 1972)

Of the three kinds of representation we referred to in Chapter 5 – observer/recorder, delegate and plenipotentiary – it is the first which a worker usually occupies when a group engages with a decision-making body. For example, it is members of the group who should speak on behalf of a delegation during a meeting. The worker's role should be much more one of helping a group prepare for the meeting. He or she must be adept at calculation, and at encouraging leaders of a group to assess, with tactical acumen, the pros and cons of different approaches before what are often very testing encounters for group members. They should also list the possible alternative stances the group might adopt, such as the following:

- *Empathising with the target.* This approach, much favoured by Alinsky, requires group members to comprehend the others' problems, without losing their capacity to present a strong case and to apply pressure. This can suggest where pressure might most effectively be applied. Political judgement can be increased, too, when a worker can distinguish the professional role or job which a person has to perform from his social role.
- *An appearance of reasonableness.* It may be sensible for a group to project a reasonable and responsible image, particularly when it suspects that the target may use alleged unreasonableness or irresponsibility by the group to discredit it.

Groups need to guard against helping authorities to ignore their case by attacking the way in which the group presents itself. Paying attention to the question of how to approach an organisation is one way of preventing that outcome.

- *Multi-focused strategies*. We indicated earlier the advantages of developing multi-pronged strategies as opposed to relying on one or two tactics. Yet there may be resistance in a group to that argument, based either on ideological reluctance to 'play the game' of mobilising forces in its favour or on a refusal to believe that more than one action arena is necessary at any one time: 'We are going to talk with the committee' – implying that that by itself will resolve the matter – can be the collective opinion of a group, and a suggestion by the worker that other action needs to be happening at the same time can receive short shrift. In this case, a worker can point to situations where groups have made effective use of multi-focused strategies from which other groups can learn.

Our survey of the skills required by community groups when they are engaged in identifying and negotiating with decision makers, and the complementary role of neighbourhood workers, has had to be selective. It is a rich area which draws not only on the varied experiences of workers but also on the practice and study of labour relations, environmental action and politics. Groups and workers will never be provided with blueprints for action in neighbourhood work. They need to develop action appropriate to their goals and to the opportunities of the situation within which they are organising. This last point underlines again the essentially political nature of the skills we have discussed.

Relating to other groups and organisations in the community

Consideration by neighbourhood workers of the value of helping to form federations of community groups and umbrella organisations is less evident than it was in the past; chiefly, we suspect, because the energies of groups and workers are now focused more on partnerships, networks, alliances and community forums. The idea itself, of coordinating the efforts of similar groups and organisations, is not new: in the voluntary sector, councils for voluntary service and rural community councils are formed on the basis of providing a focal point for voluntary organisations; in the community sector, community associations and community councils have operated on the same principle, usually in a smaller geographical area, for some time.

Neighbourhood groups can draw upon well-tried experience when they consider how to relate to other groups and organisations in the community, and there is now a useful literature about this form of organising. There is recognition of the difficulties and challenges, at the same time that it is seen to be an essential line of development for neighbourhood work. Group members will come owing prior allegiance to their own organisations and may have varying degrees of ambivalence as to the purposes of a wider association with other organisations. Such ambivalence has been experienced by many workers who have tried to form borough or city-wide groupings. An invitation will be given by workers to groups to send representatives to a meeting, yet, as in this example reported to us by a community work team: 'Quite a lot turned up, but nothing came out of it. We followed up the meeting with a questionnaire, sent round to get more details of issues important to tenants. No replies came back.' Afterwards, the worker considered that it had been too complicated an exercise, transport problems made regular communications difficult between groups in the borough, they may have been too keen to talk about problems rather than highlight what strengths and experiences people could share with each other, and there was a lack of structure of communication.

Clearly, there are crucial factors to take into account when the idea of a federation is being considered. It is important to estimate the resources of the likely constituent groups, especially the availability of committed and skilful people to work at that level. Workers must judge, too, how much existing groups will *in fact* have in common, as compared with working together through discussion and sharing of ideas. It will be the priority issues facing a neighbourhood which will be the major determinants of the form and content of organising. This becomes evident when a cluster of neighbourhoods faces either an immediate crisis or a long-term problem – The campaigning approach of London Citizens has recognised the potential of building a shared agenda, often bringing together churches, other faith groups and organisations on a borough or wider basis.

Sometimes there is an imperative to build links between community groups – for example the efforts made by networks of groups in north Belfast to negotiate with diverse communities for the removal of the high walls which, despite the peace settlement in Northern Ireland, still separated some neighbourhoods. Barry Checkoway, in an article which explores how ideas about community change and diversity, comments: 'Diverse democracy requires people who can communicate with others who are different from them, discuss concrete issues, and find common ground. Lacking this, civil society will decline' (Checkoway, 2009: 16).

We consider here how groups tend to come together across an area, and suggest that one way of understanding various experiences is to distinguish between those organisations which originate chiefly from the *practical needs* of community groups and those which form more through realisation of their *common values*. However, we shall see that the results of both these starting points tend to be similar.

It is important to emphasise that, in concentrating in this section upon federations, umbrella and similar organisations, we do not wish to imply that this is the only way for community groups to relate to each other. It is possible, for example, for groups to keep in touch through exchanges of newsletters, social media, websites and by mobile phone, and a worker needs to consider carefully the benefits of these and other options before advising groups to bind themselves together organisationally. Taking such a step is usually a major undertaking for any group, which is why we propose to examine it in more detail.

Practical origins of organising between groups

Most community groups look to either a defined geographical area or to a local authority boundary when they consider working together. Other boundaries are sub-regions and the scope of national funding regimes. Town and city-wide organisations have been formed around a range of different issues and problems.

Play is an activity which often leads to the formation of umbrella organisations. Playgroups, holiday playscheme committees and environmental projects can all frequently appreciate the benefits of joining with groups which have similar interests. It enables them to coordinate their activities, which can be particularly important when several groups share one resource such as a minibus, and it can provide an essential framework for securing future funding. Islington Play Association in north London is an umbrella organisation which campaigns for play facilities and runs a children's centre, adventure playgrounds and summer events:

> If you are running services for children in Islington, we can offer you a whole package of support. We run a play forum where you can meet other people who are working in the borough, share ideas and get answers to every day issues that come up when you are working with children and young people. We can help your management committee to understand their roles, plan the services and ensure that all paperwork is correct and up to date. We offer many different kinds of training and can put on specific sessions if you request them and we have enough people who want to do it. We also offer targeted support to play providers through our projects (www.islingtonplay.org.uk).

Many tenants' and residents' associations have also realised the practical gains they can obtain by establishing an umbrella grouping, either on a borough-wide basis or covering a smaller area, such as neighbouring estates or districts. Some associations are long-established. Camden Community Empowerment Network, also in north London, brings together and supports the voluntary and community sector in planning and decision-making within the borough of Camden.

There are, accordingly, a range of essentially practical reasons why groups seek to form umbrella organisations. Inevitably, they overlap with other motivations of group participants and workers. At the same time, it can be seen how the federated form of organisational structure can have advantages for agencies as well as for the member groups. Housing associations and local authority housing departments have found that federations can be effective ways of communicating with tenants.

As workers acquire more experience of working on environmental issues, it is likely that new forms of collaboration between traditionally separate groupings will emerge. It can happen too when whole industries are closed, or threatened with closure or large-scale redundancies: community projects can support the campaigns of trade unions and local authority-based organisations. They can also work together to access new government funding possibilities.

Implications of inter-group organising

We have referred already to the two most obvious benefits to be gained by forming umbrella organisations. First, there is increased scope for *coordination of activities* of neighbourhood groups which face similar practical problems and which have common interests. In the previous chapter, we refer to the extent that a community group develops a host of relationships with other groups and organisations. Here we underline the need for a group to build on such relationships in order to coordinate information and ideas about who can do what and what resources might be available; the relationships are communications systems as well as channels for support and exchange. They can function through *ad hoc* coalitions and formal multi-agency alliances, set up and held together through networks of like-minded individuals. Second, there is the potential for developing a *collective strategy* by groups, and the opportunity to concentrate their resources in campaigns which buttress the work undertaken by groups separately. In this sense an umbrella organisation presents an opportunity for local people to exert more power. Sometimes the saliency of an issue can mean that this way of organising starts from a low base. Coalitions can be built in response to an external threat or event:

> Its aims will generally be focused on achieving a limited goal, such as winning a policy decision, organising an event, defending or obtaining a common resource. Once the coalition has achieved its purpose it may either dissolve or transform itself into a more structured organisation that could take on the management of a service, a building or other more permanent project.
>
> (Gilchrist, 2019: 50)

We have juxtaposed two points of origin of umbrella organisations, but for each of them the outcomes and benefits from that level of organisation appear to be similar. The following are three such consequences which can become evident.

Sharing facilities or resources

Four or five active groups which agree on effective ways of relating to each other can then often decide to 'come under one roof'. In this way they reduce their individual costs, or acquire a permanent base for the first time. They can also then be in a position to offer facilities such as meeting rooms, Internet and printing facilities to all the community in addition to their existing members. The possibilities of sharing training and educational resources can be another significant consequence for groups which share common interests and problems.

Stimulation of new projects

Creation of an additional level of organising can help provide new momentum among active groups, a desire to 'have another go' at a seemingly intractable problem or to tackle something new. For example, a small federation of tenants' associations in one area of south London gave regular support to a new community health project, thereby helping a difficult scheme to make an effective start. Strong umbrella structures can have the effect both of restoring services to the community and of inspiring new initiatives.

Establishing new resources

Federations of community groups may decide to pursue new programmes or projects themselves, as opposed to putting their weight behind those of other people. A number of umbrella groups have successfully pressed for the setting-up of advice centres.

We end discussion of the federation form of organising by pointing to some of the risks and dangers associated with it. Timing is crucial. It is essential for a group to be strong in itself before it considers forming serious organisational links with other groups. This must include the availability of individuals who have the skills and time for this kind of work; the problem is that it is often the leaders of local groups who themselves come forward to participate in umbrella organisations, and the consequent burden can become insupportable. The discovery that groups with similar aims operate with very different styles, which may clash in the umbrella situation, is another risk which local groups take. Or the formation of several groups into a federal structure may release latent divisions within a community which thereby becomes collectively weaker in relation to the rest of society. It is also likely that, because they are working predominantly at a strategic and policy level, federations are open to manipulation by political parties.

The most serious danger, however, is that the federal focus may have the effect of drawing a group's leaders away from their own group in a major way; ultimately this can lead to a weakening of the group's credibility in the neighbourhood. 'Losing' leaders in this way is, in effect, another form of co-optation, particularly if the federation begins to assume responsibilities which could be said to lie with the local authority. Leaders begin by learning to be effective at a federal level, but they can end up by being able to talk only with each other, or to resource holders in other organisations. A neighbourhood worker, of course, has an opportunity to point out, when appropriate, that leaders of a community group – chairperson, secretary, treasurer – do not necessarily have to be its representatives to other organisations. Yet often it is precisely these individuals who have the energy, interest or ability to take on an additional role.

Finally, we underline the need for federations of community groups, and individuals active within them, to receive adequate support. This may not necessarily always be neighbourhood work support – strong administrative resources can often be the priority. But frequently such organisations will need to be serviced by neighbourhood workers, and their role and tasks may acquire a markedly different emphasis than when working directly with community groups.

Constituency and the general public

The connection between the activities of a community group and the whole neighbourhood must necessarily be close. In several senses, the neighbourhood provides the lifeblood of a group: it is where membership, which is in a continuing state of decline and renewal, comes from. Furthermore, community development values give significant emphasis to the need to ensure that membership of groups is kept as open as possible, and both workers and leaders should try to counteract the tendency of organisations to control who should belong to them. This is particularly important because of the extent to which groups have been drawn into partnership working with large organisations: 'Communities and practitioners need to recognise that partnerships do not necessarily hold their interests at heart and that they need to exploit them rather than be controlled by their agenda and priorities' (Pitchford, 2008: 108).

Groups can gain measurable strength by making certain they keep in touch with wider community views. In the final analysis, local residents will be their constituency. Effective public information techniques by groups (newsletters, use of digital technology, public meetings, press statements etc.) can be used to do this. The following is an example from a project on the Beckhill and Miles Hill estates in Leeds:

We have experienced many challenges and want to share what we have learned with similar groups. The Two Hills Project wants to:

- forge community links;
- explore issues and share knowledge;
- champion community concerns;
- celebrate community successes.

We want an easily accessible network that will enable us to do this and believe that an internet site is the ideal starting point for such a network. This ground-breaking community-based network will enable like-minded people to share news, advertise community events, create a local contacts directory and pool ideas.

(Two Hills Project, personal communication)

Finally, groups can never afford to forget that their own members are part of a wider community, and they need to be self-critical of the effects that being active with a group can have on their personal and family lives as well as on their relationships with neighbours and friends; for many people the political is inseparable from the personal.

It is also essential for community groups to keep a check on how their actions affect the community for less obviously functional reasons. Characteristically, only a small proportion of local residents become involved in community groups; how the 'silent majority' perceives and passes judgement upon a community group has to concern the latter's members if its work is not to be seen as irrelevant or even alien.

The idea of a group monitoring the effectiveness and acceptability of its work becomes more tangible once it is applied to an analysis of existing power and influence within a community. The cutting edge of organising can frequently only be discerned when it disturbs, or stimulates response from, powerholders or community influentials. Anticipating how they will judge community action, especially that which relates most obviously to social change objectives, must form a central part of the repertoires of groups and workers.

The significance of this area underlines again the need to have a good understanding of constituencies. If, for example, a worker perceives there to be a tenants' association in existence, which is inactive but which retains control of key resources in a community, the worker cannot consider how to handle that situation without first obtaining a rudimentary understanding of the extent of covert support the association retains in the community, and an assessment of the potential constituency for forming a new tenants' association.

Yet, while it may be self-evident that workers need to realise that neither they nor the groups with which they work exist in a political vacuum, experience suggests that neighbourhood workers have to keep working at understanding all the implications. It indicates how much more workers can learn and adapt material from theoretical and policy concepts such as those to which we refer in the opening chapter – social capital, civil society, social inclusion, co-production and capacity building.

A social policy perspective

The distinction we make between groups which move towards tackling broader issues by allying with each other, and groups which have policy questions as their central concern, cannot be clear cut. By the latter we mean essentially a long-term commitment to working on a particular problem, which has an obvious national or international policy dimension. Instances when groups come together simply for tactical reasons, and do not meet again, cannot be said to be working with a policy perspective.

Policy work does not necessarily imply that a group must join with other groups. On the whole, however, it does require a high degree of organisational strength and confidence on the part of community groups. It is possible to identify action by community groups which is either pitched predominantly at a *national/international* level, or which picks up on policy issues chiefly at a more *local* level. In the first category, we have in mind the situation where a community group or groups decide to take up a national or international issue, to put time and energy into trying to change legislation or to influence government policy. Another area is the networking and support which takes place between community groups on a global basis, making use of technology and with a commitment to supporting each other in struggles against poverty and injustice, in working for sustainable development and in learning from each other. Increasing numbers of community groups have experience of such exchanges. There has also been extensive networking among community workers and researchers, leading to the development of skills and techniques, notably of participatory learning and research methods. Forging links with interested academics who can offer advice on policy issues should be considered. It can also be worthwhile for groups to work on policy matters with national organisations, such as the Joseph Rowntree Foundation and the New Economics Foundation, which have a strong interest in action at neighbourhood level.

When one turns to action on policy questions by groups at local, city or regional levels, there is a range of experience upon which to draw. Many groups attempt to give their activities a policy perspective, but there have been a number of campaigns and programmes which stand out as having been especially concerned with the relationship between local community action and national or international policies. Not surprisingly, a high proportion of the international examples are about climate change. There are also strong links between poverty groups and organisations and between social enterprises.

It is usually very difficult for any practitioner who is absorbed in the details of his or her work, usually in contact with small numbers of individuals in a specific location, to conceive of that work relating to and frequently influencing policies. The connection to wider processes is hard for anyone to make. Neighbourhood workers are no exception.

Yet policies are not formulated within social institutions in isolation from external influences and pressures, and work undertaken by grassroots workers can have an effect on decision makers and others who are traditionally classed as having responsibility for policy formulation. It is this interpretation of policy with which we ally ourselves, and we believe that it is particularly relevant to neighbourhood work. Neighbourhood workers have a mandate which encourages them to 'fill out' social and economic policies, that is, to interpret and discuss them with local people, and also to support community groups whose aim is to implement or change policies.

Workers are right to search for ways of helping the groups with which they work to understand the policy implications of their action. This can range from discussing with a group which is pressing for a community centre the financial and management policies of education authorities to community centres, to sharing with a housing group recent developments in national housing policy; or it can range from helping a group to understand the legislation on disability to ensuring that groups are informed of opportunities to participate in policy conferences on social inclusion and regeneration.

In terms of having clear ideas and relevant information about policies, the worker can be an essential resource for a group which is developing its ideas. The worker can play a supporting role behind a group's turning towards the broader issues which do not relate obviously to a local situation but which in fact can be the determining factors of that situation. The danger to be alert to is that, in a group's involvement with broader policy issues, it does not drift away from its own constituency.

Learning to administer and provide services

The study of the administration and the provision of community-based services touch on a central question in neighbourhood work: to what extent should workers be concerned with helping groups to acquire and provide services, as opposed to facilitating social action and awakening people to opportunities for participating in, and influencing, local decision-making processes and wider social, economic and environmental issues? It is easy for both community groups and neighbourhood workers to be drawn increasingly into managing services which they have struggled to obtain. This issue has become of central importance for community groups because of two very powerful pressures on them: encouragement from government for groups to run services and public expenditure cuts. As a consequence, groups are increasingly involved in helping to preserve services. A report for the Joseph Rowntree Foundation makes this point:

> Neighbourhood working is especially vulnerable. There has been major restructuring of neighbourhood working in local authorities, with the loss of many frontline jobs. In times of recession, discretionary services are more vulnerable to cuts than statutory services. Many neighbourhood workers nationally find it hard to neatly sum up what they do, and therefore what their value is.
>
> (Richardson, 2012: 2)

We chose to include a section on administering and providing services in this chapter because the questions which it raises are of a similar order to those we have examined with regard to a group's relationship to other agencies. Opinion about a potential resource or service will tend to point a group in one direction rather than another. It is therefore useful for a worker to be able to offer some clear thinking on the matter. He or she should update themselves on co-production schemes, especially as they can provide a route towards a group's organisational stability and sustainability. If a group plans to broaden its work by, for example, joining a local, national or international network, it should be encouraged to think about ways of ensuring the continued strength of its base and avoid overstretching its resources (Richardson, 2008). The difficulty is illustrated by the range of meanings and ambiguities often attached to such phrases as 'self-help' and 'community-based' services.

Local people need identifiable skills to help them run their own organisations – if that is what they have decided they want to do – so that they have control over what services they wish to offer and how they will provide them. The neighbourhood worker always has to be alert to finding ways of helping groups acquire necessary knowledge and skills to do this. In other words, the worker has to give explicit recognition to ensuring that local needs are met in addition to undertaking the enabling and organising work that so strongly characterises neighbourhood work.

The variety of transactions which occur between local groups and resource holders suggests, however, that the reality is more complex than a simple flow of resources from those who administer to those who demand them. There are at least six ways in which community groups attempt to influence resources, and these categories of resource influence are discussed in the following. They are offered not as a rigid list but as a guide for clearer thinking on this question.

1   *Resource acquisition.* A local group achieves an increase in, or addition to, a stock of particular resources. The group and its constituency acquire resources to which it has had little or no access. The acquisition of a new community centre by a tenants' association is an example. So too is the availability of a food bank.

2   *Resource improvement.* Groups make an improvement in the quality of existing resources and services, for instance, caretaking facilities, insisting that a children's walkway is made safe, making officials more responsive to community needs.

3   *Resource rejection.* A group opposes and rejects the proposed introduction of resources to its community. Examples are provided by airport and motorway opposition groups and resistance to proposals for sheltered homes for vulnerable and stigmatised people in the community.

4   *Resource conservation.* Groups attempt to conserve existing resources in the face of a threat to remove or reduce them. Thus one group may want to restore an historic building or protect an open space while another may wish to preserve the real incomes of its members in the face of impending rent increases or reductions in welfare benefits. Community groups who help constituents to resist evictions or harassment by landlords who wish to use the property for other purposes are engaged in the conservation of a housing resource.

5   *Resource administration.* Local residents take on a contract for administering and managing a local resource (such as a playground or short-life housing) but where the resources are owned and/or financed by a housing association or the local authority.

6   *Resource provision.* Residents attempt to provide services outside and independently of the formal structure of service provision.

This conceptualisation of neighbourhood work activities relating to services offers a relatively concrete and specific way of ordering an often bewildering diversity of activities. Within each category of resource influence, these activities are seen to have features held in common throughout the fields in which community groups traditionally operate. The categorisation also helps us to see that in any one of these fields community groups are attempting to influence decisions about resources in a variety of ways.

What can we learn from experiences of the categories of administering services and providing them? We identify four areas:

Mutual benefits

Dealings between an action group and its target over resource administration and provision may be effected through collaboration because they are transactions that often carry benefits for the target, for example, a housing association acquires management and administrative resources when residents agree to the setting up of an Estate Management Board, while residents acquire new organising experience in addition to more control over local resources. This mutuality of benefits is often overlooked or thought unimportant as agencies struggle to respond to the change proposals of community groups. Agencies can be aware of negative factors like hostile exposure by the media, irritated councillors and inter-agency tensions. Their attention often needs to be drawn to advantages which accrue to them as a result of community action, and this can be most evident when groups are administering or providing services.

Human resources

Different people may be better suited to some kinds of transactions than to others. For instance, residents who work effectively in a community group concerned with resource improvement or administration may not work as effectively with transactions about resource acquisition and vice versa; many local residents who fight for a housing cooperative will not be as interested and effective in administering it. This is not to deny the motivation and capacity of local people to change and develop through learning new skills. We are talking about a gradation of effectiveness, not a rigid categorisation. Many local people have gained enormously from helping to run local services, in terms of political awareness and control: parents who run playgroups and go on to undertake training, or advice centre volunteers who become adept at representing individuals at tribunals, for example.

The shift by a group to administration or provision of services also offers an opportunity to counter a tendency for a group to be over-dominated by a few individuals. Organisational structures established for this purpose may not always succeed. The identification of new tasks and responsibilities can represent, as it were, a break with the past and enable new leaders to come forward.

The injection of new blood into the active leadership of a group may sometimes require open challenge to be made to the existing leadership if it is seen to be ineffective, autocratic or is simply considered to have 'held the reins' of power and authority for too long. There may be conflict here between the qualities and predispositions of individuals who come forward to engage in service provision or administration and the qualities and personality needed to challenge entrenched leadership. We suggest that this is because the former is a less controversial area than, for example, struggles to acquire or reject resources, and it may therefore attract people who lack sufficient will or ability to question the position of established leaders.

Workers employed by community groups

The advantages and disadvantages of neighbourhood workers being employed by community groups remain widely discussed. We do not know the number of such workers at present but it will not be insignificant.

There are the inevitable administrative tasks for a group which face any employer: payment of salary, arranging tax, insurance and pension, and so on. It is essential for a group to have an able, experienced and trusted person who can be responsible for this work, and there should be an awareness by the group of its seriousness. 'Moonlight flitting' by treasurers of groups occurs rarely, but there have been bad experiences where administrative jobs have not been maintained, or where communication between an employed worker and his or her employer has broken down. In the long term, the ability of a group to sustain reliable working conditions is as good a test as any of its capacity to run a service.

Careful thinking by a group of the support networks required by a worker should run parallel to strong administration. As a group gives consideration to this question, a range of key topics will emerge: a *support group* for the worker which can offer guidance and advice about details of the worker's programme; the opportunity for the worker to have regular meetings with a *consultant* or with a peer supervisor; ensur-.ing that attention is given by the group and the worker to the latter's *training* needs and aspirations; encouraging the worker to *network* with those doing similar jobs across a wider area than the neighbourhood where he or she is based. Such meetings, combined with informal opportunities to discuss and share with colleagues, could either provide additional stimulus and support or be a forum for debate and joint action on common issues. Sarah Banks suggests that the concept of critical practice is underpinned by the idea of a community of practitioners: 'The opportunity to discuss, debate and agonise with colleagues is a vital part of keeping critical practice alive and the critical practitioner motivated and supported' (Banks, 2007: 148).

We have only listed key areas to be considered by a group concerned to offer effective support to a worker. Despite the work involved in establishing them, any community group which wishes to keep its staff and run an effective service will need to address itself to them as thoroughly as any other agency should do.

Finally, we draw attention to a critical area for workers employed by community groups. Broadly, this turns upon the maintenance of political compatibility between a worker and his employer. The classic question of worker accountability is usually debated in the context of a worker and a large bureaucratic organisation, traditionally a local authority. In one sense the question becomes redundant when a worker is employed by a neighbourhood group – there is no other body to which the worker could be accountable. It would be more accurate, however, to argue that the question has to be reinterpreted in the situation we are discussing. Tension between a worker and his employer can arise over disagreement either about strategies, objectives, methods or working conditions, or about values and ideology. Even when employed by a group, the worker may feel he has accountability to other groups or to people who are not organised.

Worker role and problems

There is little doubt that the area of administering and providing services draws upon a different range of skills on the part of a neighbourhood worker to those he or she uses in most other situations. The advantages of a project or an agency having a clear idea of the knowledge and skills it wants from a worker become apparent here. It can be unrealistic to expect one person to work with groups engaged in a wide variety of resource transactions.

A project which can employ a team of workers is at an advantage, for tasks can be shared among staff members according to their abilities and interests. There can be wisdom in rotating some tasks directly to do with service provision. This can avoid a situation developing where one worker becomes trapped into helping to provide a service, such as a resource centre, because local people are not yet able to run it themselves. Changing the worker can prevent one person from becoming frustrated and can also indicate to sponsors and local people involved that reliance upon a full-time worker will not continue forever. There is also a strong case for neighbourhood workers to concentrate on 'signposting' to people information about available services, thereby protecting, to an extent, their own facilitating role and the time and energy of community group members. Keeping this focus for neighbourhood work also retains the scope for encouraging groups to be as inclusive in their membership as possible. This theme is discussed by Patience Seebohm and Alison Gilchrist in their study of community development and mental health:

> There was general agreement among community development practitioners, their community participants and mental health practitioners that they have an important role in enabling people with mental ill-health to live equally respected lives alongside others without distinction. They sought to help staff across public services, voluntary sector and private sector understand distress as something we all experience in some form, and as something we all can help to address. Community development practice aims to create the kind of communities and services which promote well-being and reduce stress.
>
> (Seebohm and Gilchrist, 2008: 52)

'Signposting' in this way can be undertaken equally effectively for other services such as help with jobs, training, playgroups, health and housing.

Our discussion in this chapter of both how a group relates to the rest of the community and of the topic of service administration and provision illustrates again how workers need to be able to move easily between roles during different phases of the neighbourhood work process. It is essential to retain flexibility and versatility. This receives further emphasis from our analysis of endings in neighbourhood work in the final chapter.

References

Banks, S. (2007) 'Becoming critical: developing the community practitioner', in H. Butcher *et al.* (eds), *Critical community practice*, Bristol: The Policy Press.

Brager, G. and Specht, H. (1973) *Community organising*, New York: Columbia University Press.

Bunyan, P. (2010) 'Broad-based organising in the UK: reasserting the centrality of political activity in community development', *Community Development Journal*, 45, 1: 111–27.

CESAM/SABO. (2000) *Neighbourhood democracy at work*, Stockholm: SABO.

Checkoway, B. (2009) 'Community change and diverse democracy', *Community Development Journal*, 44, 1: 5–21.

Gilchrist, A. (2019) *The well-connected community: a networking approach to community development* (3rd edn), Bristol: The Policy Press.

Hunjan, R. and Pettit, J. (2011) *Power – A practical guide for facilitating social change*, Dunfermline: Carnegie UK Trust.

O'Brien, C. (2007) 'Integrated community development/conflict resolution strategies as "peacebuilding potential" in South Africa and Northern Ireland', *Community Development Journal*, 42, 1: 114–30.

Pitchford, M. with Henderson, P. (2008) *Making spaces for community development*, London: CDF.

Richardson, L. (2008) *DIY community action. Neighbourhood problems and community self-help*, Bristol: The Policy Press.

Richardson, L. (2012) *Working in neighbourhoods, active citizenship and localism*. Online. < www.jrf.org.uk> (accessed 18 May 2012).

Seebohm, P. and Gilchrist, A. (2008) *Connect and include. An exploratory study of community development and mental health*, London: National Social Inclusion Programme in association with CDF.

Von Hoffman, N. (1972) 'Finding and making leaders', abstracted in J. L. Ecklein and A. A. Lauffer (eds) *Community organisers and social planners*, New York: Wiley.

11 Leavings and endings

The closing phase of the neighbourhood work process is often one of apprehension and difficulty for both workers and group members; yet a search of the literature for advice and understanding about this phase shows that little has been written by or for neighbourhood workers about the various forms of ending. There is also a dearth of material in related fields such as group work and adult education, though what has been written about endings in group work is relevant to the neighbourhood worker.

Endings may *seem* less important and demanding (i.e. until the worker is experiencing one!) than the other stages of neighbourhood work such as making contact with local people and helping them form and run a community group. These earlier phases may be viewed as substantial parts of the work while endings *seem* to be something that occur after the action and are, by implication, therefore less important. This is, of course, untrue because some endings occur during the earlier phases of the work when, for example, the worker decides to leave or a group falls apart. Another reason why theorists and practitioners may give less attention to endings is that endings are bound up with a number of intense feelings experienced by the worker and the group members – feelings of loss, separation, sadness and guilt as well as pride, satisfaction and solidarity. Endings, too, are inextricably connected to the beginnings of other things: workers and members invariably end in order to begin somewhere or something else, and the demands of a new situation will usually be sufficiently strong to prevent the outgoing worker from dwelling upon the ending of his or her work.

The inability to deal adequately with the problem of endings may also be understood by the strong wish, even fantasy, among many in community work to see action in the community as something that has no ending. The Biddles, for example, see community work as a 'non-terminal' continuing process, and one can discern in the thinking of Alinsky and his community organising successors the idea of the steady growth of a group that links up with a wider social movement, through networks of

DOI: 10.4324/9781003310006-11

people's organisations. Those who stress process or educational goals in community work often seem to believe that individuals and groups move on from task to task, reaching higher and more general levels of understanding and influence. The fact that this rarely happens does not seem to diminish the wish that it *should* happen, and it may be the strength of this wish for permanent activism that distracts attention from managing endings.

Leavings and endings are often linked to failure. It is of interest that the phrase about ending that is most common in community work – 'the job of the community worker is to put herself out of a job' – assumes success on the part of the worker and the local residents. But endings are as often brought about by *lack* of success and progress, either on the part of the worker or of the group. Failure, and the endings associated with it, is often something difficult to contemplate.

Endings that are brought about by the withdrawal or departure of the neighbourhood worker may be facilitated where the worker has managed to keep the dependency of the group on herself at a fairly low level. The more dependent a group has become on a worker, the harder it will be to manage the worker's leaving and its own affairs after her departure. One of the core skills in neighbourhood work is to provide support, help and resources to a group without this fostering an overdependence of the group on the worker. Yet the need to keep dependence at a low level strains against the equally important need for the worker to 'get close to the group'. Most neighbourhood workers may be seen as outsiders in the communities they work in, by virtue of their education, lifestyle and ambitions. Thus most workers have purposefully to build up their relationships with local people, and to communicate their identification with them. It is no easy task both to get close to a group, provide it with support and help and at the same time to foster its independence.

Evaluation

Evaluation becomes of central importance in leavings and endings. We explain in Chapter 2 why evaluation has to be an integral part of all stages of the neighbourhood work process but it is during leavings and endings that report writing and dissemination come to the fore. As we have seen, there has been a sea change in attitudes towards evaluation, both within organisations that support community development and amongst practitioners. There is now a significant literature and accessible evaluative studies. Neighbourhood workers and community groups will need to be highly active in ensuring that messages from evaluation are communicated and listened to. Equally important is the consolidation of knowledge and learning gained about the process of doing neighbourhood work and the performances of the worker, organisations and residents. This is the point at which evidence of learning, social capital, capacity building, community cohesion, empowerment and participatory democracy can be brought together, analysed and disseminated.

Types of endings in neighbourhood work

Endings in neighbourhood work occur in a variety of ways, and we propose to analyse them according to whether they happen to the group or are initiated by the worker.

The group comes to an end

A common type of planned ending occurs when a community group accomplishes its goals. In some cases, this will mean the physical breaking up of a group that has, for example, sought rehousing for its constituents. More common, perhaps, is the case where a group achieves its goals (or, on the other hand, recognises that they cannot be achieved), and the members decide that it is more appropriate to dissolve the group than to work on new issues. However, its members may remain informally in touch with one another and some may also join other community groups or come together at a later stage to take action on a neighbourhood issue as members of a newly formed group.

A group may also come to an end, first, because it has decided to amalgamate with another group with similar aims and constituents (e.g. the amalgamation of two neighbouring tenants' associations, or that of two pressure groups) and, second, because it has run out of the funding necessary to continue its operations.

Another kind of ending for a group (though it is not strictly an ending) occurs when a group makes a significant *transition* in the nature of its activities. Transitions of this kind have to be prepared for and managed by worker and group as diligently as real endings, and should involve rites of passage that formally recognise and facilitate the transition experienced by the group. There are a number of such transitions in community work. For example, a group that has succeeded in *acquiring* a new resource in the neighbourhood like a youth club has to face the transition to *managing* the resource and, as we discussed in the last chapter, this will make different demands on the time, knowledge and skills of its members. A group that has achieved its objectives may decide to stay together and pursue a new set of goals that relate to a 'new' need in the area that perhaps its previous work has unearthed. Groups which have their funding cut may seek to become social enterprises in order to generate income through trading or providing services. And a group may decide to work solely through a larger federated organisation of community groups. This is the kind of 'larger nucleus group' identified by the Biddles through which a smaller group makes the transition necessary for dealing with wider community, city and regional issues. This matter was discussed in Chapter 10.

The experience of a group in a rural part of Hungary demonstrates how it is possible to plan ahead:

> We should not forget about fatigue or death. To keep the organisation alive it is essential to ensure that there are successors. An organisation that is not prepared to do so will risk disappearing. Ever since we started, we have provided space and opportunities for our young people to learn, gain experience and practice. We tolerate mistakes in our spaces but you have to take responsibility for those mistakes. We see that some young people who have come to us make use of what they have learnt, here and elsewhere as well. They are committed to professional innovation and leadership. Besides them, there are others who are more rooted here – they are the ones who undertake the day-to-day activities and provide a solid foundation for our work. However, to keep our processes sustainable, we always need renewal, which we hope will come also from the returning, well-travelled and experienced young people.
>
> Eva Monostori, coordinator (personal communication)

So far we have identified a number of ways in which endings in neighbourhood work occur in a planned manner. Naturally, the corollary of an ending that is planned to take place is that both worker and group will have to deal with feelings and emotions about the ending, and carry out tasks that prepare for that ending and its consequences. In the later part of this chapter, we shall look more closely at these feelings and tasks. While many of them are generic to the different types of planned endings that we have discussed, it is also true that each type of ending will make different demands on the worker and the group.

But endings also occur unexpectedly. By their nature, unplanned endings almost always constitute, or revolve around, a crisis in the life and work of a community group. The premature ending of a group may come as a shock and surprise to its members, but the factors that lead up to and bring about such endings may often be discerned by members and worker in advance of the ending. Sometimes group and worker can cope with events so as to avert or postpone the ending; at other times, group and worker feel powerless to intervene to arrest the dissolution of the group.

There seem to be four kinds of developments through which unplanned endings occur.

1   There is a sudden and extensive loss of the group members or its leaders. Such a loss may occur in a variety of ways, including mass resignation of officers and key members, the withdrawal of support by the group's constituency or the failure of an annual meeting to elect a new committee. Conflicts between members are an ever-present possibility in groups and can lead to splits and eventual collapse.
2   Groups in which officers have carried the burden of the work may break up if those officers suddenly are unable to carry out their duties because, for example, of illness or rehousing.
3   There is a gradual loss of membership, and the group withers away despite the work of some group members and the worker to reinvigorate the group and attract new members. Gradual loss of membership may occur because of apathy, slow progress and lack of interest in the issue pursued by the group. Also, people may become deterred from remaining or becoming members of a group if they believe that to do so would jeopardise their interests.
4   There is a crisis in the group precipitated by the death or serious illness of a key person.

Unplanned endings such as these pose particular problems for the worker, not least feelings of guilt that the events that led to the endings might have been averted or foreseen if the worker had been more skilled, or less harassed by demands from other groups and from his or her agency. The worker has to decide whether to put time and energy into starting the group again, or whether it would be better to move on to some other issue or group. A worker who believes it is right to help to start the group again, and is encouraged to do so by local people, then has to face, together with the rump of local people who remain, other decisions about the goals, activities and procedures of the re-formed organisation.

The prospect and the actuality of the ending of a community group are likely to cause a variety of emotions and feelings in the group members. The reason for the ending of a group will naturally determine the kinds of ways in which the members experience ending. The premature ending in crisis of a group is likely to leave its members disillusioned, with feelings of failure and a wariness of collective action that may make them reluctant to join a community group ever again. On the other hand, the ending of a group that has successfully achieved its goals will leave its members strengthened and confirmed both in their personal abilities and in the efficacy of collective action.

Even when the work of a group comes to a successful conclusion, the feelings of achievement of its members will be tempered, and may be over-ridden, by feelings of uncertainty and loss – loss of the support and friendship found in the group, and loss of the opportunities for creativity, helping others, responsibility, authority and status that were present in the work of the group. For many members, the group will have had a major impact on their lives, affecting their family and work, and many will ask the question, 'what now?' If the work of the group becomes less and less demanding as ending approaches, members may encounter the kind of emptiness in their lives that they fear when the group eventually breaks up. Thus the prospect of ending will provoke a welter of ambivalent feelings amongst the members and, as we shall discuss later, it is the task of the worker to help the group 'work' on these feelings and understand the kind of effect they may be having on the day-to-day business of the group.

The neighbourhood worker decides to leave

The decision of the worker to end or reduce the association with a community group is the occasion for quite a different type of ending. There are a number of ways in which this can occur.

The worker decides to move to another job

This nearly always involves the worker leaving her agency and ceasing to work in the area in which the community groups she has worked with are located. There are diverse reasons why a worker will move on to another job, including the desire for change, better work prospects and a more congenial agency setting. In some cases, a worker may decide to leave an agency as a result of a disagreement with supervisors about the activities of a group and the worker's relationship to it. There are various possible ways in which a group and the outgoing worker can manage this situation.

- The outgoing worker seeks to hand over the work to her successor and, with the consent of the group(s), introduces the successor to the people she has been working with. Adequate record-keeping is essential in facilitating an effective handover of work. The worker may also suggest to the group and the agency that local people are involved in the selection of the successor. The *way* in which the incoming worker is introduced to the local groups can be a major determinant of her future relationship with them. The different levels of care and attention that a new worker may experience in being introduced are captured in the following extract from a new worker's records sent to us from a project in south London:

> With Ogden House, I developed a relationship with individual committee members before attending my first meeting. This was especially the case with the chairperson who took it upon himself to introduce me to the project patch as well as to the Ogden House situation. With Leighton Street playground, however, I was catapulted straight into a committee meeting

without first having had the chance to meet individual members. The difficulties caused were compounded by the fact that Joan [the outgoing worker] came late for the meeting and I was not introduced to anyone until the meeting had finished. I then experienced considerable difficulties in getting to talk with the chairperson, though I did easily manage to meet other committee members before the next meeting.

There is value in the new and outgoing worker holding joint sessions with the local people with whom they work because if the old worker enjoys a good relationship with the group, she can help legitimate the new worker.

- The outgoing worker hands over responsibilities to a local person, who has been trained and prepared in anticipation of the worker's departure. This indigenous worker may be an unpaid local activist or a resident employed by a local group(s) that has managed to raise money to employ a community worker.
- A local organisation such as a council for voluntary service undertakes to support the group.
- The group joins a federation or coalition of other community groups.
- The group decides to carry on without another worker, and without seeking help from local agencies, though it may use them for specific resources and information.

Each of these arrangements for carrying on after the worker's departure has its own costs and benefits, and these need to be assessed in the light of the particular needs and circumstances of each group.

Finance for the worker's activities comes to an end or is withdrawn

This situation is 'built in' to those community work projects that come into a neighbourhood for a fixed period, say three or five years. But in other circumstances, withdrawal of funding for projects may, unfortunately, be on a much shorter time scale and often unexpected. An example from Tallaght, a town on the outskirts of Dublin, brings home the sense of shock and disappointment for residents and staff even when there has been a review and appeals process:

> After some 20 years in existence, both Tallaght projects were obliged to make staff redundant, transfer their work to the local Partnership and close their doors within weeks. The reasons for the decision of the department were both baffling and abrupt. Completion of objectives was one reason, duplication of work was another. Not a shred of tangible evidence was provided to back these conclusions but a contention that their work could be adequately carried out by Dodder Valley (formerly Tallaght) Partnership was offered as a final reason.
>
> (Lloyd-Hughes, 2010: 101)

Similar situations have happened in the United Kingdom as a result of public expenditure cuts. Local authorities and other statutory bodies are being starved of resources and, unfortunately, neighbourhood projects and neighbourhood workers have been easy targets for cuts.

As we shall discuss later, part of the worker's tasks may be to help the group(s) to raise money to employ their own staff. Withdrawal of funding can also lead a worker to identify with a group potential new sources of income, notably through the setting up of a social enterprise.

The worker remains in his job, agency and neighbourhood but believes that the time has come to end or reduce activities with a particular group – or his agency has decided to assign him elsewhere

The worker or agency may reach this decision because they believe that other groups in the neighbourhood are in greater need of the services offered, or that the group is now able to function either without the workers' help or with reduced involvement so that he becomes merely someone who provides specific resources and information. He may decide either that the group no longer needs the kind of contribution he has been making, or that if it does, it can either provide it from amongst its own members or seek it from other people in the area, either local people or other professionals.

This kind of withdrawal by the worker from an ongoing group may be handled in one of the two ways. First, there is the time-centred approach in which the worker has made it clear from the first contact with the group that he will be withdrawing after a certain time such as 18 months or two years, though the worker indicates he will be flexible about the exact timing of the withdrawal. The advantages of this method are that the reality of the worker's leaving is always clear to the group and that it may increase their motivation to achieve their goals before the worker leaves. Such a contract about withdrawal can also include the possibility of a worker saying he will *partially* withdraw at the end of a time period, and be available thereafter on an occasional basis.

The second approach is more goal-centred and has two variations. In the first, the worker makes it clear to the group from the start that she will withdraw when the group has achieved certain goals. These goals may be agreed upon by worker and group. The advantage of this variation is that it appears less arbitrary than using time to determine withdrawal, and the worker leaves the group when its morale and confidence should be high as a result of achieving its goals. A possible drawback of this approach is that the group may 'put off' attaining its goals in order to hang on to the worker; also, it may not be possible to achieve agreement between the worker and the group about whether the goals have been achieved.

The other variation of this goal-centred approach occurs when the worker comes to a decision that the goals have been reached, or that the group is well on the way to achieving them. The worker's assessment of the group's progress, and her decision to withdraw, are, so to speak, sprung upon the group – there was no contract or understanding from the outset of the action that the worker would make such an assessment and consider withdrawing. The worker's decision may be made public, in which case she informs the group of the decision to withdraw, or private, in which case the worker assesses the group's progress and begins gradually to drift away from it, becoming less and less involved in its activities. Clearly, a disadvantage of this second variation of the goal-centred approach is that the worker's 'sudden' announcement of withdrawal may affect the group's progress towards the goals in question. And no matter how well the worker explains the decision and reasoning behind it, there is a good chance that her motivations will not be fully understood by the group who may be left feeling let down and rejected.

Whichever approach is used – time- or goal-centred – the worker will feel uncertain and apprehensive about the rightness of the decision, and the validity of the criteria used in setting the time and goal boundaries. No matter how confident the worker is in the autonomy and resources of the group, she will still worry about whether the group 'can manage without me'. In particular, the worker will be aware of limitations that exist on the autonomy of the group. Residents take part in community groups in their spare hours, with limited time and energy at their disposal. They may be unlikely to develop the knowledge, skills, resources and contacts of a full-time worker, and they will not have access to the kinds of resources that a worker may exploit in her own agency. The outgoing worker will also wonder about the group's strengths in being able to deal with conflicts and problems arising within the group – disagreements and rivalry, for instance, about policy, money and leadership. Though the worker and the group may be confident about how the group has learnt to tackle issues and deal with problems in the past, they may be less certain about the group's ability to generalise what has been learnt and to apply such learning to new situations that arise in the future. In addition, both worker and group may be apprehensive about how well the group will identify the resources it needs to carry out its tasks, and how able it will be in acquiring those resources.

The group that faces the prospect of losing its neighbourhood worker will experience a range of feelings, including, again, a sense of loss. A group, too, may feel guilty – believing it made too many demands on the worker, or that the worker lost patience with it. There may possibly be a sense of failure if the members think that the worker's departure signals a lack of faith and confidence in them. It is important to note that such feelings and fantasies about losing a worker may characterise even the most independent and successful of groups. If the worker stays on in the neighbourhood to help other groups, some members of the group from which she is withdrawing will feel slighted, unimportant, rejected and envious of the other groups with whom the worker will be in contact.

Apprehensions about the future may also appear in the group as the day for the worker's withdrawal approaches. Members will privately and publicly voice their fears that without the worker they will not be able to deal with the problems that will crop up in their work. Indeed, in the last period of association with the group, the worker can expect to encounter two phenomena that may be seen as unconscious 'ploys' to persuade her from leaving. The first is a series of crises in the life and work of the group – about, for example, leadership bids or money – that are 'designed' to show the worker that the group is not ready to function without her; and second, officers will 'contrive' to carry out the tasks of the group with less confidence and skill than characterised their work in the past in order to demonstrate their felt inability to carry on the leadership of the group without the support and advice of the worker. Needless to say, these negative feelings and fears will coexist with feelings of achievement and expertise, and of independence of the worker.

The experience of endings

There are a number of ways in which groups manage their feelings about the ending of a group, or the withdrawal of a worker. Our experience suggests that conflicts between committee and constituency, and disputes within the committee about the behaviour and decisions of the officers, are common behaviours in community groups facing termination. There occurs, too, a denial of the impending reality of the ending and groups will try to 'postpone' the ending by:

- becoming inefficient in their business through absenteeism, lateness, forgetting to bring papers to meetings and to follow up on decisions made at meetings,

and becoming more lax about decisions about the time, place and purposes of meetings;
- looking around for other issues and problems to take up, no matter how inappropriate;
- becoming reluctant to carry out and complete their tasks;
- moving into being friendship and solidarity groups.

Some members may find their anxieties about ending are so hard to bear that they unconsciously want to 'end' before the end of the group. They will perhaps cease to attend meetings and behave to all intents and purposes as if the group's work were complete, or become involved in disputes in the group that threaten to accelerate its termination. This may go hand in hand with attempts to disparage the work of the group and to refuse to acknowledge both what individual members gained from the group and its success in achieving its goals.

We conclude this section by summarising the kinds of reaction to termination that Garland *et al.* (1972) stated 'have been observed repeatedly in groups which were in the process of termination. They are devices typically employed by members to avoid and forestall terminating, on the one hand, and to face and accomplish it, on the other'. The six basic reactions are:

- *Denial.* This is achieved in two ways. First, members may 'forget' about termination, and appear surprised when the worker draws their attention to it. Second, members deny termination by 'clustering' together to form a 'super-cohesive' group.
- *Regression.* Members backslide in their ability to deal with interpersonal and organisational tasks. Disagreements and quarrels may erupt, particularly directed against the leadership and the worker. The group may also revert to the levels of functioning that were characteristics of its earlier days.
- *Clinging.* The members will deal ineffectually with the group's business, or bring up new problems for the group, because there will be a feeling that the worker will stay on, or the group will continue, if the members can demonstrate the need.
- *Recapitulation.* The group will throw up demands to review and even repeat experiences and events that occurred in its formative days.
- *Evaluation.* Recapitulation, particularly through review sessions, may lead the group into discussing the value of the group's work and the experience of the group by individual members.
- *Flight.* There are two kinds of flight. The first is a 'destructive reaction to separation' in which the members will deny any positive experiences gained in and from the group. The second form is more constructive and members attempt to 'wean' themselves from the group by developing contacts and interests outside the group. The new contacts, which may be started well in advance of termination, serve to substitute for interests and gratification which will no longer be fulfilled after the group's end. They also represent a broadening and maturing of interests and skills.

So far we have discussed some of the kinds of ways in which group members may experience endings. We now turn to look at the feelings of the neighbourhood worker. He, too, is likely to have made close and satisfying relationships with people in the group, and in its constituency. He will have invested his skills, energy and time into helping the group form, develop and achieve its objectives. He will have struggled with the group through periods of decline, low morale and conflict when the possibility of achieving anything may have looked remote. It is not surprising, therefore, that a worker facing the end of a group or his own withdrawal will also experience some feelings of loss, as well as those of pleasure in noting the progress of the group towards independence and goal achievement. The days before termination/withdrawal are, for the neighbourhood worker, a period in which he will reflect upon, and evaluate, his contribution to the work of the community group, analysing and learning from the good and bad aspects of his interventions. This kind of self-evaluation is likely to be linked to the worker's attempts to anticipate the kind of challenges he will face in his next job or assignment.

The worker may feel anxious about the quality of his work with the group, and inevitably he will feel that he could have done more. The events in his work that he sees as failures will loom large, perhaps overshadowing that which he has done well and conscientiously.

His worries about the quality of his work may be exacerbated if he falls prey to assimilating the group members' own sense of failure and disparagement which, we have noted, may characterise their feelings as the termination date approaches. The worker who is leaving for another job may also experience some guilt if he is looking forward to leaving, and if he is leaving in order to go to a 'better job' with more pay and responsibility. He may wonder whether his own self-advancement is being achieved at the expense of the progress of the community group. Alternatively, a worker who has been made redundant by his agency and who has not found another job may feel depressed and unmotivated to sustain involvement with the group.

The worker who is withdrawing from, or reducing her services to, a group in order to work with others in the area may be apprehensive about the rightness of her assessment of the group's competence. She will want to be sure that her reasons for withdrawing are really what she thinks they are – she must be certain that she is withdrawing because the group no longer needs her contribution and not because she wants to escape from problems and difficulties encountered in working with the group. She must then manage her worries about whether the group will continue to cope without her, and form some confidence that the gains made by the group are relevant and likely to endure in the work it faces in the future.

Finally, we must consider that the worker who is changing or losing her job and leaving the community altogether will be leaving behind far more than the people she has worked with in the particular community group(s). First, she will have feelings about leaving those – probably other professionals – who have worked with her in supporting the neighbourhood group, and – if she is leaving voluntarily – she may wonder whether they construe her leaving as a desertion and a lack of commitment to the group and the area. She may feel guilty at leaving them 'to carry the can', and apprehensive about their ability to support the group alone and the effect of their different values and approaches on the work of the group.

Second, the worker may be leaving her colleagues in her agency or community work project. Assuming she is leaving the agency on good terms, she has to manage her sense of loss of colleagues and friends. In particular, her seniors and colleagues are likely to express some remorse that they have not done more in relating to the worker's activities, and in providing adequate support for the worker. It may be that in some agencies the departure of the first neighbourhood worker to be appointed to the staff signals the completion of an innovation or experiment, and staff members have to consider whether to appoint another worker. This agency assessment of the worker's contribution is yet another aspect of the period of evaluation that occurs in the termination of work.

The tasks involved in endings

It should be clear from the discussion that both the community group and the neighbourhood worker have to carry out certain tasks in order to prepare for, and finally achieve, the ending of the group or the withdrawal of the worker. Ending is a phase in the life of a group or relationship that has to be worked upon just like any of the other phases in group development.

A familiar distinction in the group work literature is that between the phases of pre-termination, termination and post-termination. We shall use these phases (though using different words to describe them) to consider the tasks facing the group and the worker in endings.

Before the ending happens

In this phase, there are four tasks to be carried out: evaluation, disengagement, stabilising achievements and administration.

Evaluation

Here, using a planning and evaluation framework as discussed in Chapter 2, the task of the neighbourhood worker is twofold. First, she must help the group to evaluate its own experience and achievements, partly in order to help members achieve the kind of recognition and reinforcement of their progress that will promote confidence in themselves when the worker has left, or when the group finishes. Second, the worker must encourage some evaluation by group members of her own contribution to the group. This is done partly to see how far the worker has achieved the goals outlined in her initial agreement with the group, and partly as an aid to the group in planning the resources it will need in the future. Identification of the kind of contribution made by the worker will better enable the group to assess if it can now make that input from within its own members, if it is still needed, and what resources it will need that have to be obtained from outside the group. The worker may need to foster such evaluation with individual members of the group and with the group in one of its own committee sessions. Achieving an effective balance between private and public work is one of the skills of carrying out the pre-termination tasks.

In specifying the aforementioned tasks, it is important to reiterate the key message of Chapter 2 that evaluation needs to run through all stages of the neighbourhood work process. Here we are referring to a final evaluation which builds on evaluative work that has been undertaken before.

Disengagement

The most important task of the worker is to help the group acknowledge and confront the reality of ending and then to help members openly to discuss their attitudes and feelings. As we have already noted, there may appear in a group a number of behaviours that seek to deny or forestall the fact of termination, and the worker must be able to recognise these and use them to encourage the group members to admit the reality of ending and to prepare for it.

The worker must introduce the subject of ending or withdrawal early enough for the group to work positively on it, but not so soon that people's feelings about termination serve to inhibit the achievement of the group's goals. His purpose in encouraging openness about ending is to ensure that felt but unexpressed emotions do not negatively affect the work of the group in its last period or the relationship between people in the group. Again, it is important to note that the worker will probably have to work with individuals and the group in this task of disengaging from relationships with the group. The worker who is leaving a group may be tempted to discuss his leaving only with individual members of the group (and, perhaps, only the officers). But even if all the group members know of his leaving and have discussed it with him, there is every reason to encourage the members to discuss the issue as a group. His leaving is, after all, a group problem, and it is the group that will need to discuss how they will prepare for his leaving and the period afterwards.

The other aspect of the disengagement of relationships is the worker's attempts to reduce his involvement in the affairs of the group. This will typically be the concern of a worker who is withdrawing from the group or who is leaving to take up another job. What the worker has first to accomplish is a willingness in himself to let go; he must then decide upon the speed and timing of his steps to reduce involvement. There are no general prescriptions to help him in this task for he must take into account the particular circumstances of the group he is working with. He must also decide whether his decision to reduce his involvement is a private one, or whether it is one he will share either with a group's officers or with the group as a whole. Again, he must decide this on the basis of his knowledge of the group and the nature of his relationships with its members. Some openness about his interventions may be desirable, however, for group members will inevitably soon perceive the ways in which he is cutting down on his involvement. The risk that the worker runs in concealing his intentions is that group members may misinterpret his reduced involvement as a rejection of themselves, or as a lowering of his commitment to them and their work. Both these perceptions may adversely affect the work of the group.

There are a number of ways in which the neighbourhood worker can detach himself from a group in anticipation of his withdrawal or departure. They are as follows:

- reducing the number of committee meetings of the group that he attends;
- being present for only part of meetings by arriving late or leaving early; a worker may arbitrarily decide how long to be at a meeting, or to be present only for some agenda items and not for others;
- contributing less and less to discussion during meetings of the group;
- absenting himself from the informal, but highly important, meetings of some group members that frequently occur before and after committee meetings;
- reducing attendance at meetings that the group holds with other groups and organisations;
- deciding not to get to know new members of the group who join in the period before his leaving;

- introducing new resources to the group – other professionals or his successor as a neighbourhood-based practitioner;
- reducing social contacts with group members.

The worker who is housed in an accessible neighbourhood base like a community centre may also decide to stay away from the base for a period each week. This absence will help to reduce his availability to group members and facilitate other tasks he has to carry out before his departure, such as the writing up of his records.

Stabilising achievements

The worker's concerns in this task are to make sure that positive changes and gains will be maintained after he is no longer involved. The worker seeks to leave the group feeling confirmed in its abilities and reasonably confident about meeting the challenges that lie ahead. This is achieved partly through taking opportunities with group members to assess the work of the group, and explicitly to recognise the progress that has been made by the group and by individuals within it. But chance, too, plays a part in this stabilisation process and the worker might hope in the period before her withdrawal/departure that no real crisis (as opposed to those manufactured by the group to persuade the worker to stay on) or heavy demands will appear to test the group's confidence and perhaps to undermine it.

In addition, there are a number of things that the worker may consider doing to stabilise and strengthen the community group. These may include:

Working with the group to discuss whether it wishes to make use of the services of the worker's successor, if there is to be one. The group may also want to discuss with the worker whether it will be participating with the agency in matters like preparing a job description, interviewing and selection. A neighbourhood worker in a project that has come to the end of its grant and is closing down might also work with a group, or federation of groups, to obtain funding and other resources like office space to employ its own staff. If this is successful, then further work must be done with the group in coming to a decision about what kind of staff it wants, the work they will do, and the kind of arrangements that are necessary for advertising, interviewing and selection.

Ensuring with the group that its structure and procedures are as stable as possible for the tasks that lie ahead. The group's constitution, and its arrangements for dealing with finance, the election of officers and the recruitment of new members, might be reviewed at this stage.

Discussing with other outsiders and professionals the nature of their continuing contribution to the group after the worker has left. The worker must ensure that they relate directly to the group and see the need for remaining available to the group as resources. She must ensure that these other professionals do not see themselves as relating to the group through herself because if they do, their association with the group may fall away after she has gone. The idea of a low level of continuous 'light touch' support, explored in an analysis of the Joseph Rowntree Foundation's Neighbourhood Programme, is relevant here:

> The programme was able to demonstrate the potential of a small pot of flexible funding, a little mentoring from a trusted 'critical friend' and the opportunity to meet with other neighbourhood organisations across the three countries (Wales,

Scotland and England) – at a cost of roughly £7,500 per neighbourhood per year. In neighbourhoods that experienced poverty and fragmentation but were not targeted by a regeneration programme of some kind, this was often the only means of support.

(Taylor *et al.*, 2007: 9)

Additionally, the worker may discuss with the group what new resources, if any, it will need in the future, and the identification and acquisition of these resources will be part of her work in the pre-termination phase. There may be a danger in introducing new resources, particularly new members, in the pre-termination phase. While new members are necessary, it might not be the best time for them to be given responsibilities within the group, for if they fail (through lack of experience and skills, for instance) this might lower morale and confidence in the group at a time when it needs to be as strong as possible. The neighbourhood worker perhaps needs to discover whether, in the pre-termination phase, a group can cope with and tolerate newcomers; a worker who thinks that it can must help the group assimilate and welcome them without giving them too much initial responsibility. The primary task in this phase is, after all, to build upon and consolidate what the existing members have learned and achieved.

Clarifying with service agencies in the neighbourhood the nature of their continuing relationships, if any, with the group. This would include indicating to agencies the kinds of resources they have available that might be needed by the group.

Clarifying the extent to which the worker will be available after the date of her departure/withdrawal, and agreeing on the kinds of issues which it might be appropriate for the group to bring to the worker. The nature of availability is a difficult decision for the worker; besides constraints on her time, the worker will not want to agree to any arrangements that she suspects will foster the dependence of the group on herself. On the other hand, the worker will not want to give the impression that she does not care about, or is not interested in, the continuing fortunes of the group. Neither will she want to appear to intrude upon the efforts of her successors in establishing relations with the group. At the very least, the worker may want to leave a contact number – although the danger is that the number may not be available to new members who join. This could lead to situations in which the worker is being consulted by one faction in a group, and not by the other. Her picture of events is then incomplete.

The worker may also seek to make other kinds of arrangements for keeping in touch with the group. For example, she may ask the group to send her its minutes, newspaper clippings, reports and so forth, and express her interest in attending group events like fund-raising occasions, social outings and the annual meeting. She may, too, want to remain in touch with other professionals and service agencies in the area who could pass her news and information about the work of the group.

In seeking to clarify the nature of her availability after the group ends, the worker must bear in mind that group members will have formed their own views about it. It will be part of her task to openly discuss with people both her and their expectations about future contacts. The failure to do so may result later in uncertainty on the part of group members and the worker, and feelings of disappointment, rejection and resentment.

Helping the group develop and consolidate its relationships within the wider community. This is, of course, particularly important for members of a group that is ending because it has completed its tasks. Members may need support and advice in finding elsewhere the opportunities they found through membership of their group. Particularly important for members may be alternative sources of friendship, support and outlets for creativity and continuing involvement in civic affairs or community action. Likewise, the worker may need to assist an ongoing group to make the contacts with other organisations in the community that might be useful in pushing forward the future work of the group.

Administration

The fourth set of tasks for the neighbourhood worker in the pre-termination phase may be seen as basically administrative and relating more to his agency or project than to the group(s) with whom he works. Because the worker is likely to be very busy in the period before he leaves, these agency-based responsibilities may tend to get pushed aside in favour of time put in with group members. There seem to be five important administrative tasks for the worker.

1   *Writing up records and preparing reports on the work.* The worker will need to complete this writing in order to facilitate the orientation of his successor to the work, to have available a set of recordings from which he and his agency may evaluate the nature of his work, and to guide and influence the agency in its future development of neighbourhood work. The worker may also want to prepare papers for dissemination or publication that illustrate what he sees as important issues and ideas that have arisen from his work.

2   *The evaluation of his work with his agency supervisor and colleagues.* Evaluation is important not least because professionals in public service must attempt to assess how effective they have been in achieving their goals, but also because it is a learning experience from which the agency can benefit in the drawing up of proposals for the employment of another practitioner to replace the one who is leaving. The worker should also learn from evaluation things that will be helpful in his future practice, particularly feedback from the agency about how he has worked as a colleague and change agent within the agency. The worker, too, can give feedback to his supervisor and to the agency in general about the nature and quality of the support for his work that he has experienced. This kind of evaluation is essential if a worker and his agency are to develop in their practice and management of neighbourhood work and other forms of community-based practice.

3   *Effecting closure on his relationship with agency colleagues and those in other agencies with whom he has worked.* Such closure is too often confined to informal social events, but there is a need to create opportunities for the worker to discuss his work with his colleagues inside and outside the agency. Such discussions might be based upon papers prepared by the worker about the different aspects of his work.

4   *Clarifying with his agency what is to be done about appointing a successor.* This may involve making the case for the continuation of a neighbourhood work appointment because other staff may press to use the post to employ another type of worker; hence, the effective evaluation of his work will have an important influence on whether the agency continues to employ a neighbourhood worker. The worker might also seek to clarify what role local groups will play in discussions about appointing a new worker.

5   *If a neighbourhood worker is not going to be replaced, ensuring that the agency will still provide some kind of support for community groups.* In situations where funding both for neighbourhood work posts and community projects has been cut, raising the question of future support will undoubtedly be challenging. If a worker has, over a period of time, won the respect of one or more senior managers, this would be the time to urge them to address the issue of long-term support for community projects. Mobilising sympathetic councillors should also be considered.

The ending

At the point of termination, the neighbourhood worker's main task is to ensure that the group gives itself what Baldock has called a 'decent burial'. He writes:

> There is a great danger that people will be left feeling that the experience was not worthwhile, that 'it's useless trying to start anything around here'. It may be valuable for the group to wind up formally with an appreciation of what it has been able to achieve, quite apart from the fact that the existence of funds may make a formal dissolution necessary. But the burial should be a decent one.
>
> (Baldock, 1974)

The ending of a group may be formally achieved through a meeting that makes arrangements about the disposal of funds and what is to be done about dealing with correspondence and other issues that might occur, and through some organised social event like a party or outing that marks the ending of the group. The literature on group work emphasises the importance for termination of some ritual or closing ceremony that helps members make the final acknowledgement of the ending of the group. It has been suggested that activities that help towards marking the fact of termination should be guided by three major principles: first, they should indicate and confirm the success of the group; second, they should be activities and events that reduce the cohesiveness of the group, and thirdly, activities should help members to consolidate their attempts to reach outside the group. Some workers have been embarrassed (but perhaps inwardly pleased) by some of the events arranged by community groups to mark ritually the departure of the worker or the ending of the group. The worker may be formally given a gift at the last meeting, or made the subject of speeches of gratitude at farewell parties.

After the ending

We have already noted that the worker and group members may have a variety of social and/or work contacts after the event of a group's ending or a worker's departure or withdrawal. Additionally, the worker may renew contact with group members if she has written up her work and she wants their comments on her drafts.

Conclusions

We have endeavoured in this chapter to indicate that leavings and endings have to be thought about and planned for, just like any other phase in the process of practising neighbourhood work. They must be managed effectively, not least because a group member's experience of the ending of a group will be an important influence upon her or his attitude towards engaging in collective action in the future, or in feeling confident enough to place neighbourhood issues in a broader social, economic and political context. If first impressions count, last impressions linger, and the neighbourhood worker should do all she or he can to avoid unhappy endings overshadowing the positive aspects of the group's activities.

References

Baldock, P. (1974) *Community work and social work*, London: Routledge & Kegan Paul.

Garland, J. A. *et al.* (1972) 'A model for stages of development in social work groups', in S. Bernstein (ed.) *Explorations in group work: essays in theory and practice*, London: Bookstall Publications.

Lloyd-Hughes, J. (2010) 'Relevance and redundancy: the contribution and discarding of community development projects in Tallaght', *Working for Change: The Irish Journal of Community Work*, 2: 102–7.

Taylor, M., Wilson, M., Purdue, D. and Wilde, P. (2007) *Changing neighbourhoods: the impact of 'light' touch' support on 20 communities*, York: JRF. Online. Available HTTP: <www.jrf.org.uk> (accessed 5 April 2012).

Appendix

Evaluating neighbourhood work – Case study

The following case study illustrates how the approach to planning and evaluation described in Chapter 2 can be used to inform neighbourhood work. The example is imaginary but based on a town in the west of Scotland.

Susan is a neighbourhood worker in Northside. She was appointed through an area regeneration partnership, with a remit to encourage networking and community building. Northside is a regeneration area with a population of 2,000 people. It consists of a mixture of high-rise flats, maisonettes and houses. The hub of the area is a bleak, windswept shopping mall that contains a local services centre which houses meeting facilities, a community café, youth drop-in centre, library, local learning centre and a gymnasium.

For much of her first six months in post, Susan talked with local people, to understand how the circumstances of the neighbourhood impact on people's lives. These conversations have confirmed that Northside suffers from a range of social, economic and health problems. Unemployment is high, poverty is widespread, housing conditions are relatively poor and there is a high turnover of tenancies. Associated ill health is also apparent, and educational performance and access to further and higher education is low. Drug misuse is fuelling criminality and community safety is a significant issue. The area is physically isolated from the rest of the town and transport costs are high. All these factors reinforce the negative image of the area. There are few community groups and organisations in the neighbourhood and they are largely inactive and unrecognised, by both local people and public service providers.

Susan has concluded that she should seek to encourage more active community groups to form, and to begin to focus attention on addressing some of the problems in the area. These are the general outcomes that she has identified, and are consistent with her job remit and the aims of the partnership. In talking to residents, several women had protested about discarded needles being found in the car park at the back of the shopping mall. They had described this as a symptom of the increasing risk from drug dealing and misuse in their community. They were particularly fearful for their children, not only due to the drugs themselves but also from increasing violence and the risk of being drawn into criminality. Susan decided that she should give priority to working with this group, because it would be consistent with her role and aims, and because the women had asked whether she would be able to help them.

The neighbourhood worker brought together the women who had expressed concerns and encouraged them to discuss with each other how they felt about the drugs problem, how it affected them personally, and what they thought about its impact on the neighbourhood as a whole. Through these discussions, the women got to know each other better and realised that they had much in common, not least the desire to do something about the problem, and the recognition that they could take an initiative. They formed an action group and decided to call themselves 'Women Improving Northside' – or WIN.

A closer relationship with Susan was also fostered, as it became clear that she was able to help focus discussions, bring in information and describe the various organisations with an interest in drugs issues. She also had an ability to offer support and contacts. Through these discussions, and with her support, WIN established and agreed the outcomes they would wish to see, and the indicators they would use to ascertain whether the outcomes had been attained. While Susan did not use the language of 'outcomes' and 'indicators' with them at first, she did explain their meaning and purpose such that the group itself began to use the language in due course. The resulting outcomes and indicators were recorded on flipchart paper, and later written into a simple table as follows:

The project should achieve these outcomes	*Outcome indicators – how we would know things had changed*
A safe community where their children are free of the risks of the drug trade	Recorded drug-related crime reduces. People say they feel safer walking in the neighbourhood at night.
The opportunity for enjoyable and worthwhile activities for young people	WIN collaborates with others, e.g. establishing links with Northside youth club and joining their campaign for a skate park – helping both groups to achieve their outcome.
Growth in confidence and skills	WIN applies for and carries out a community-led research project. WIN is invited to present its research findings to the Alcohol and Drugs Action Team (ADAT) and does so effectively.
Capacity to plan and take action together	WIN applies for and carries out a community-led research project. WIN supports the Northside youth club campaign.

The first two outcomes could be seen as 'task' outcomes: concrete changes in the quality of life, while the others can be seen as 'process' outcomes – of value in themselves but also necessary for the task outcomes to be achieved. It may also be noted that despite the focus being on a single issue, outcomes could be expected in relation to several other concerns in the neighbourhood.

Having agreed the outcomes sought, Susan initiated discussion with WIN on how best to take things forward. This involved identifying the main interests in the issue, and considering their motivation, capacity and opportunity to support or challenge the group.

Motivation

For Susan and the regeneration partnership there is a commitment to building the capacity of the community to address local needs. This is congruent with national priorities and the local community development strategy. There is also a commitment to tackling drug culture and its consequences for community safety. The community and WIN are motivated by anger about threats to the safety and welfare of children, fear of dangers to children and adults, and their ambition for a safe, attractive, positive community. They also enjoy working with others to achieve change. Several public services, including the police, health agencies, schools, children and family services, and community and voluntary organisations are also likely to be motivated to help, as the drugs issue is of concern to them.

Capacity factors

Susan and her colleagues have skills and experience in capacity building, access to resources including an operational budget, equipment, access to specialist advice and managerial and policy support. The community is likely to be able to commit time, energy, resilience in the face of adversity, self-organisation skills, the ability to highlight the threat locally, and the emerging confidence and self-belief necessary to tackle the threat. Other agencies would have the capacity to offer time, knowledge of drug-related issues, skills and resources to tackle drug abuse problems, access to advice and information materials, as well as to funds for community activities and community health programmes.

Opportunity factors

Opportunities recognised by Susan include the shared interest of other potential partners in tackling drug misuse, and the heightened sense of crisis indicated by spontaneous protests. For the community, they include positive support from the community development team, the interest expressed by other potential partners, a positive response from the local press and the high profile of the issues in national and local policy. From other agencies interested in drug misuse came the potential to work with a locally driven campaign, improve services and increase effective partnership working and community engagement.

Resistance factors

Drug suppliers and dealers are likely to resist the action in order to maintain their power and income, and are likely to be actively resentful and potentially threatening. They might use or threaten violence, in order to exert a hold over drug users and use their resources to promote and extend the drugs market. The opportunity to address such resistance may lie in the desire for change among users, and among passive community members. Drug users would not only be likely to resist a potential loss of access to supply but may also be motivated by personal desire for change. Some agencies may be resistant due to fears of the consequences of the confrontational style of the women's group. They may resist through use of professional power and authority, and control of access to resources.

Having spent some time working with Susan on these analytical tasks, WIN developed a more complete understanding of the workings of the drugs issue in Northside, and how they might best respond to it. They also had a better understanding of how they could mobilise support and influence to focus attention on the issue, and were thus better placed to plan effectively.

As the first step in planning, Susan explored with the group the resources that would be readily available to support their efforts. Again these were recorded on flipchart paper and then written up as a table:

Resource	Source
Time – 1 day per week (attendance at group meetings, regular contact with group members to provide advice, information and training, help with funding applications, meetings with other partners)	Neighbourhood Worker
£250	Internal budget
Production of minutes/publicity/information materials	Administration
Training manuals/programmes	Good practice manuals
Training course on council premises free of charge for the women's group	Venues
Attendance at WIN's group/sub-group/office bearers meetings; training; engaging with partner agencies; meetings with local councillors/MP	Time of neighbouhood worker and WIN members
Time – attendance at community/public meetings and events	The wider community
Time – attend three meetings of group to provide information and advice on tackling drug misuse	ADAT

Discussion also identified further resources that might be needed but which would require effort to secure:

Possible need	Possible source
Meeting place	Local Community Centre – £45 monthly let
External funding	£5,000 small grants funding to carry out group activities including research, community surveys etc.
Councillors	Time – attend monthly group meetings and meetings with partner agencies as appropriate
Grant support	Support local grant application
MP	Time – initial meeting, review of group minutes/research findings, advocacy of group's issues and work in Parliament
Police	Time – attendance at group meetings/community events, provision of statistics/advice/information
Youth club	Time – attendance of youth worker and young people at monthly meetings, funds to build a skate park

Having established the resources (or inputs) to hand, Susan then turned to working with WIN to plan how to go about achieving the desired outcomes. Each proposed activity was tested for feasibility and do-ability, and the likely effect of the action on the desired outcomes was considered. This helped them to consider a range of options before deciding how to proceed. Each option could be tested on the basis of whether it would be necessary, and whether it would be sufficient, to achieve the outcomes sought.

The plan that emerged was designed as a three-stage process, with each stage being dependent on the success of the previous stage. The table shows the links between the inputs or resources, the processes or methods, and the outputs or specific actions to be taken. It also assigned specific responsibilities and timescales to each action.

Inputs/resources	Processes/methods	Outputs/specific actions
Stage 1: Neighbourhood Worker (Susan) Women's group (WIN) The wider community ADAT Meeting place	**Stage 1:** Outreach Information Acquiring resources	**Stage 1:** Susan will meet with women's group to discuss issues and actions and support them to make contact with neighbours, residents and other community groups. Susan will provide information about action that other community organisations have taken about drug issues. ADAT will be asked to provide information about drug misuse and services and ongoing advice. WIN, supported by Susan, will apply to the Big Lottery Fund for funding to carry out investigation into attitudes to drug misuse in the community and local services and actions that could be effective at community level. Timescale: 12 weeks Evaluation at 12 weeks
Stage 2 All those listed in stage 1 plus: Big Lottery Fund	**Stage 2** Capacity and confidence building Investigation	**Stage 2** Susan will work with WIN to identify, audit and where necessary develop, specific skills they may need to take action on the identified issues. If application to the Lottery is successful this will be supplemented by specific research skills support from a research mentor. WIN will conduct its research project and prepare a report on potential actions. Timescale: from sixth week to nine months Evaluation at nine months
Stage 3: All those listed in stages 1 and 2 plus: Councillors MP Police Community Safety Forum Youth Forum Children and Families Services Health agency	**Stage 3:** Campaign planning	**Stage 3:** Using evidence gathered and supported by the neighbourhood worker the group will prepare a campaign plan. This will include identifying key influencers (e.g. MP, councillor, Divisional Police Commander), considering how best to put over information they have gathered and deciding how to build community support and involvement and how to engage the interest of service providers.

Inputs/resources	Processes/methods	Outputs/specific actions
	Campaigning	Meetings arranged by group, discussions held, reports distributed, lobbying conducted.
	Networking and resource development	WIN will develop and sustain contact, and where possible collaborate with others with a shared interest in achieving the outcomes.
	Evaluation, reflection and learning	Evidence of progress against intended outcomes will be recorded by WIN and Susan and reviewed at the end of each stage of the action plan. Timescale: actions from 9 months onward: evaluation every six months thereafter

Monitoring

The lead role in achieving change was taken by the WIN itself, and it was agreed that they would co-ordinate monitoring of the action plan. Supported by Susan, they would do this by using the minutes of their meetings to record all action points that would be required to implement the action plan. At each meeting these actions would be reviewed to ensure that progress had been made on the tasks identified. Any evidence of progress against the intended outcomes would be recorded in the minutes.

Evaluation

WIN agreed that their work would be evaluated at the end of each key stage. The evaluations of progress would be based on the records kept by the group and observations and records of other stakeholders – the other organisations with an interest in the issue. At the end of stage 1, the key stakeholders were WIN itself, Susan and Gerry, the worker from ADAT who was providing advice and support. In stage 2, when they were successful in getting Lottery funding, their research mentor, Cathy, also became an active stakeholder. As they moved into stage 3, the campaign phase, they established a collaborative relationship with the Community Safety Forum and the Northside youth club, who also become active stakeholders. They were still seeking to influence others, including the MP and councillor, the police, health board and Children and Family Services. Initially, these individuals and organisations were not actively involved as stakeholders, but by the end of stage 3 they, too, were on board.

By the end of stage 1, WIN had not achieved any of the end outcomes it was seeking. They had, however, established a positive working relationship with Susan and Gerry that enabled them to acquire a better understanding of drugs issues and the kinds of responses that community organisations can make. They had also applied for Lottery funding to investigate attitudes to drug misuse in their community. They recognised that these were necessary preliminary actions and they were satisfied that they were in a stronger position to move forward. For Susan, there was evidence of the process outcomes that she was seeking. The group was demonstrating its continuing commitment to learning about drugs issues, showing that it could access and use resources and beginning to show competence in planning and taking action together.

By the end of stage 2, WIN had still not achieved any of the end outcomes it was seeking. However, the group had run a skills development programme with Susan's support, successfully obtained Lottery funding, developed members' research skills and carried out a community-led research project. All of these things demonstrated that the process outcomes prioritised by Susan were being achieved. Cathy, the research mentor, was also able to identify the capacity-building outcomes that the programme sought to achieve. WIN was increasingly self-confident, well organised and resourceful. Susan encouraged them to recognise and value these process outcomes, because they improved the chances of addressing the core problem of drug dealing and misuse. Whilst the underlying problem remained, the women in WIN felt that the activity had been worthwhile. They had not set it as an outcome but the fact that they were no longer feeling helpless in relation to tackling the drug issue was seen as valuable. They were also pleased that they have been able to provide support to the Northside youth club campaign for a skate park. Such collaboration directly with young people acting on their own behalf was an unexpected outcome.

By the end of stage 3 of the action plan, WIN had established a good working relationship with the MP and the local councillor, who were both supporting their campaign. The MP raised questions about drug policy in Parliament. The group had also established a good working relationship with the Northside youth club. Prompted by the political support for the group, the police, health board and social work department were all now meeting regularly with the group. The group had also been invited to be represented on the community safety forum. An unexpected outcome was that several of the leaders of WIN became well-known public figures, regularly interviewed in the press and consulted by service agencies. But another unanticipated and negative outcome was that they have also been threatened by drug dealers. Worrying as this was, it did suggest to them that they might be beginning to have some direct impact on the drugs trade. The threats prompted higher profile police action and residents were expressing the view that the streets felt safer. Police statistics were beginning to show a decline in recorded drug crime in the area. By this stage, WIN was seeing direct evidence that its primary outcomes were beginning to be achieved. However, the police reported increased drug-related incidents in other neighbourhoods, which might mean that the problem was being displaced rather than being resolved.

WIN and the other active stakeholders were now looking to further stages in their action and were asking the question 'what will we need to do now?' They recognised that they needed to retain attention to the original intended outcomes but widen the campaign to the whole of the town. The network of stakeholders with commitment to the outcomes originally formulated by WIN is now extensive and involves policy, programme and project levels. A new action plan is to be developed through the Community Safety Forum on behalf of the Community Planning Partnership. Whilst WIN welcomes this, they also fear loss of their own identity and 'edge' and have decided that they also need a plan for their own independent actions.

This case study underlines the importance of using planning and evaluation throughout the neighbourhood work process. By doing so, the worker and her agency were assured that intended improvements in the neighbourhood were taking place or, if they were not, provided some insight into why this was the case. Perhaps more importantly for a book that is essentially about improving practice skills and confidence, a robust approach to planning and evaluation is invaluable to the practitioner who wants to understand the impact of what she does and how she does it, and to continuously develop her craft. If she is doing this, the community will also benefit: there will be a clear recognition of progress that is being made, greater insight into the pressures affecting the community and how to address them, and greater accountability of the worker to the community. LEAP stands for Learning, Evaluation and Planning and of these it is the learning which ultimately is the most important.

Useful resources

Action with Communities in Rural England
www.acre.org.uk
Citizens UK
www.citizensuk.org.uk
Community Development Alliance Scotland
www.communitydevelopmentalliancescotland.org
Community Development Cymru
www.cdc.cymru.org
Building Communities Trust Wales
www.bct.wales/
Community Foundation Wales
www.communityfoundationwales.org.uk
Community Development Journal
www.academic.oup.com/cdj
Community Health Exchange
www.chex.org.uk
Community Practitioners Network
www.corganisers.org.uk
Community Sector Coalition
www.cscoalition.co.uk
Community Work Ireland
www.cwi.ie
Countryside and Community Research Institute
www.ccri.ac.uk
Directory of Social Change
www.dsc.org.uk
European Community Development Network
www.eucdn.net
European Community Organizing Network
www.organizeeurope.org
Faith-based Regeneration Network
www.fbrn.org.uk
GoWell, Glasgow
www.gowellonline.com
Groundwork
www.groundwork.org.uk

International Association for Community Development
www.iacdglobal.org
Irish Community Development Journal
www.irishcommunirtywork.com
Joseph Rowntree Foundation
www.jrf.org.uk
Locality
www.locality.org.uk
National Lottery Community Fund
tnlcommunityfund.org.uk
Neighbourhood networks
www.neighbourhoodnetworks.org
New Economics Foundation
www.neweconomics.org
Scottish Community Development Centre
www.scdc.org.uk
Online Progressive Engagement Network (OPEN)
www.the-open.net
Scottish Community Development Network
www.scdc.org.uk
Urban Forum
www.urbanforum.org.uk
Visioning Outcomes in Community Engagement (VOiCE)
www.voicescotland.org.uk/voice

Index

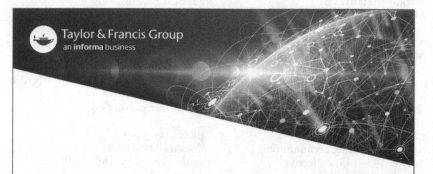